TOTAL RECALL

Mnemonics for Medical Students
Anatomy
Biochemistry
Physiology

Third Edition

DISCLAIMER

The content of this book is meant for only medical students and doctors. Non medical persons may not read this book. The mnemonics in this book are written only for the benefit of medical students and not intended to offend or harm anyone. However some people may still find a few mnemonics offensive. If you're easily offended by references to male/female anatomy, then this book is not for you and you are free to choose not to read any further.

Some mnemonics in this book are very old and well known in the medical community. I have chosen to add them to this book only for the benefits of the medical students.

TOTAL RECALL

Mnemonics for Medical Students

Anatomy Biochemistry Physiology

Third Edition

Manoj K. Khemani
MBBS, D. Ortho, FOR (UK)

Vinita Khemani
MBBS , DGO (Cal)

PEEPEE
PUBLISHERS AND DISTRIBUTORS (P) LTD.

TOTAL RECALL—Mnemonics for Medical Students

Published by
Pawaninder P. Vij and Anupam Vij
Peepee Publishers and Distributors (P) Ltd.
Head Office: 160, Shakti Vihar, Pitam Pura
Delhi-110034 (India)

***Correspondence Address:* 7/31, First Floor, Ansari Road Daryaganj, New Delhi-110002 (India)**
Ph: 65195868, 23246245, 9811156083
e-mail: peepee160@yahoo.co.in
e-mail: peepee160@rediffmail.com
e-mail: peepee160@gmail.com
www.peepeepub.com

First Edition: **2006**
***Third Edition:* 2015**

ISBN: 978-81-8445-171-9

My Parents

who taught me that every thing
is possible in life if you
work sufficiently hard enough

Preface to First Edition

Dear Friends !

First I would like to thank you for your overwhelming response. Entrance exams keep getting tougher every year. To help you crack them I am bringing you this second edition of the book with lots and lots of new mnemonics . A lot of new diagrams have been added to help you remember with visual memory. Many of the old mnemonics have also been revised. I sincerely hope you will gain a lot by reading this book.

Manoj K Khemani
Vinita Khemani

Preface to Third Edition

Dear Friends !
Our medical books are full of complex charts, tables, lists and confusing terms. One has to work very hard to remember these small but important things. During the examination it is very frustrating to find that you are getting confused or forgetting things which you had spent hours in learning. Unfortunately the PG exams are very unrelenting in this matter. A single mistake can snatch a good seat from your hands and you can lose the subject of your choice. I have very sincerely tried to present here a set of mnemonics which will help you to get that extra edge over other students, required to excel in the exams and certainly help to avoid gross mistakes.

Some students asked me: "Why bother to remember a Mnemonic when I already so many text books to cram?"

My reply: Mnemonics are not text books. The sole purpose of mnemonics is to ensure that you DO NOT FORGET WHAT YOU READ.

- Since ages, mnemonics are known to be the most powerful memory tools.
- Spending a little time over a good mnemonic can help you **retain 100%** of whatever you read!
- **No more confusion** during exams. Everything is at your fingertips.
- It is seen that students tend to spend most of their time trying to relearn what they have forgotten. You can **save a lot of time** in revision by the help of a simple mnemonics.
- Mnemonics create a strong impression in your brain. It is possible to **recall them even years later**!
- There is a common misconception that mnemonics are useless things and it is a waste to spend time on them. Believe me, by the time you finish half of this book you will realize how wrong you were.

This book is nothing like any other book on mnemonic you have seen till now.

The mnemonics in this book are arranged subject wise and system wise for your convenience. Also, I have tried to include references to the topics as much as possible from standard books. A few important topics have been discussed in details. In the end I have included some commonly asked questions in various exams, which will also help you to revise the mnemonics.

Besides being excellent for those in their MBBS this book will be immensely useful for medical students preparing for their PG entrance exams.

Best of luck for your exams.

Manoj K Khemani
Vinita Khemani

Acknowledgements

A special thanks to my teacher and my ideal Dr.Sumer Sethi (MDRD – Lady Harding Medical college) whose 100% cooperation led to the publication of this book.

Without his sincere efforts this book wouldn't have been possible.

To Dr Amrish Kr. Jha, (MBBS, RGMCH, Kolkata) who contributed a lot to this book.

To all my teachers, seniors, colleagues and juniors of Bankura Sammilani Medical College for supporting me and helping me become what I am today.

To the many anonymous contributors who provided some excellent mnemonics for this book.

Last but not the least, thanks to the publisher, Mr. Pawaninder P. Vij, Peepee Publishers and Distributors (P) Ltd., New Delhi for his full co-operation and support.

HOW TO USE THIS BOOK

- Read not more than 10-15 mnemonics every day. Too many mnemonics in a day can confuse you.
- Revise the same day and while going to sleep.
- Discuss with your friends.
- Try to recall from your memory next day. Read again if required.
- Note down the mnemonic beside the relevant topic in your textbook.
- Once the mnemonic anchors in your mind revise it mentally whenever you are free.
- Do not forget to read the relevant topic in the textbook. (A mnemonic is of no use if you don't know where to use it !).
- Revise once before exams. Stun your examiners.
- All the best.

If you have any suggestions and comments for this book please mail me at drkhemani@gmail.com . I sincerely believe that there is always scope for improvement.

Do you think you have a great mnemonic to share? Mail it to me at drkhemani@gmail.com

References

BDC	BDC anatomy – 3rd Ed
AKD	A. K. Dutta anatomy – 3rd Ed
G	Ganong physiology – 20th Ed
L	Lippincot – biochemistry - 3rd Ed
Red	Reddy – Forensic medicine - 17th Ed.
AP	Anantnarayan Panikar – microbiology-6th Ed.
R	Robbin's pathology 7th Ed.
KDT	K.D. Triphati - pharmacology - 5th Ed.
Park	Park – PSM – 17th ed.
AY	Ajay yadav – Anaesthesiology - 2nd Ed.
Dutta	Text book of Obs. by Dutta 4th Ed.
Shaw	Shaw's text book of Gynae 13th Ed
H	Harrison's medicine 16th Ed.
OPG	O.P.Ghai – pediatrics 6th Ed.
NA	Neeraj Ahuja - psychiatry - 6th Ed.
LB	Bailey & Love – surgery 24th Ed.

Contents

1 Anatomy

I. SUPERIOR EXTREMITY

1. Rotator Cuff Muscles [BDC-I-73]

<The **SITS** muscles >

Anti Clockwise from top:

a. **S**upraspinatus
b. **I**nfraspinatus
c. **T**eres Minor (not major)
d. **S**ubscapularis.

Imagine that a baseball player suffers a *'minor'* injury to his rotator cuff muscles. As a result he **'SITS'** out for the rest of the game.

☑ This cuff gives strength to the capsule of the shoulder joint all round except inferiorly.

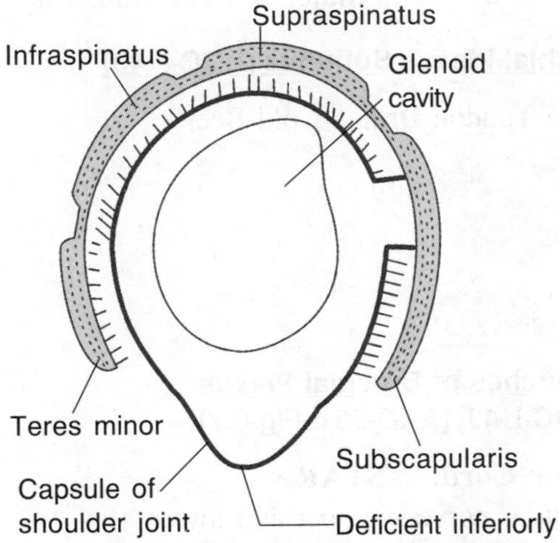

Fig. 1.1: The musculotendinous cuff (Rotator cuff) of the shoulder

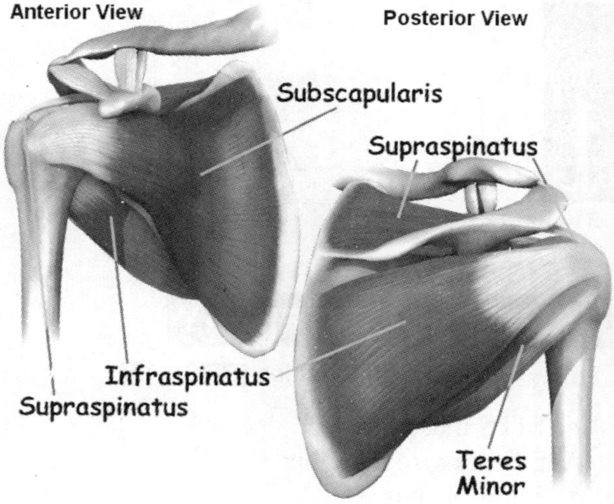

Fig. 1.2

2. **Bicipital Groove: Attachments of Muscles Near it [BDC-I -13, Fig.-2.6]**

<The **Lady** between 2 **Majors**>

Teres major attaches to medial lip of groove.
Pectoralis major to lateral lip of groove.
Latissimus Dorsi (Lady) is on floor of groove, between the Teres Major and Pectoralis Major.

3. **Brachial Plexus Subunits [BDC-I -43]**

<**R**avina **T**andon **D**rinks **C**old **B**eer>
Roots
Trunks
Divisions
Cords
Branches.

4. **Branches of Brachial Plexus [BDC-I -43] [AKD-50 c-Fig-6.7]**

Posterior Cord: <STAR>
Subscapular nerves—upper and lower
Thoracodorsal nerve
Axillary nerve
Radial nerve.

Medial Cord: <M$_4$U> or <**M**oney **M**akes **M**any **M**en **U**nhappy>
Medial branch of median nerve.
Medial pectoral nerve.
Medial cutaneous nerve of arm.
Medial cutaneous nerve of forearm.
Ulnar nerve.

Lateral Cord: <**L**ady **D**octor **S**ays: **N**ever **L**ove **M**en with **M**oustache>
Lateral cord has …
Dorsal scapular nerve—From root C5
Supra scapular nerve—From upper trunk
Nerve to subclavius—From upper trunk
Lateral pectoral nerve
Musculocutaneous nerve
Median nerve.

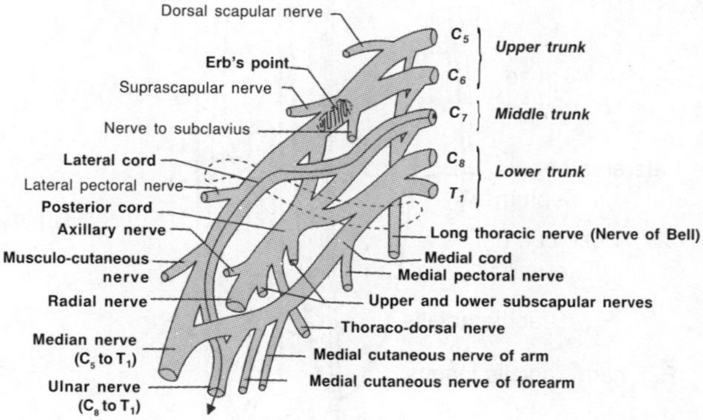

Fig. 1.3: Brachial plexus and its branches

5. Radial Nerve in the Arm Supplies [BDC-I -90, 79]

<The **BABES**>
Triceps
Brachioradialis
Anconeus
Brachialis—(lateral part)
Ext. carpi radialis longus

Supinator—(via. Posterior interosseus nerve).
Alternatively: <**A B**ody's **BEST** muscle>
(Fig. 1.4)

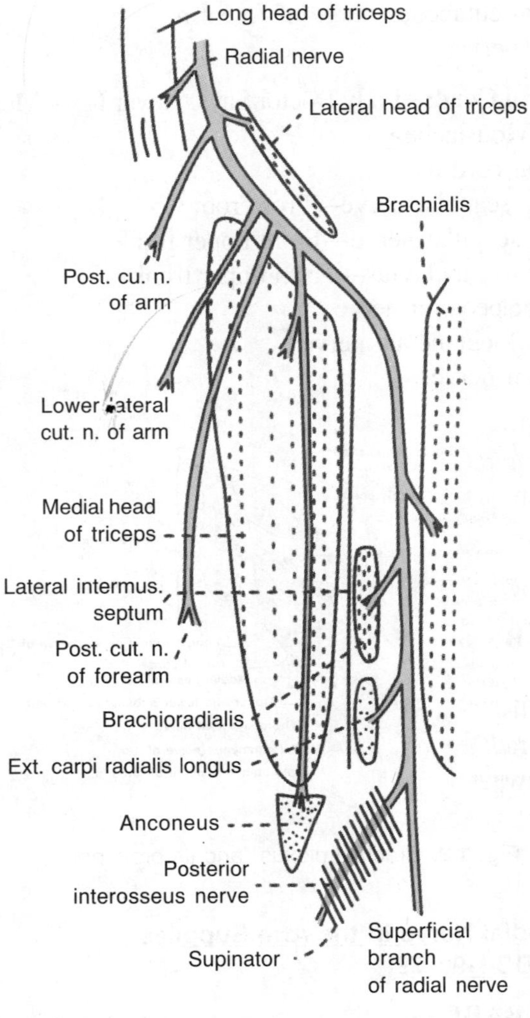

Fig. 1.4: Scheme to show the course of the radial nerve in the arm. The oblique part represents its course in the radial (spiral) groove

6. Brachioradialis: Function, Innervation, One Relation, One Attachment [BDC-I- 125]

< **B**rachio**R**adialis >

Function: It's the **'Beer Raising'** muscle, flexes elbow, strongest when wrist is oriented like holding a beer (mid prone position).

Innervation: **'Breaks Rule'**: It is a flexor muscle, but innervated by Radial nerve. (Radial nerve usually is for extensors: Recall "The BABES" rule: B was for brachioradialis).

Attachment: Attaches to **'Bottom of Radius'.**

Important relation: Behind it is the Radial nerve in the cubital fossa.

7. Muscles of the Front of Arm [BDC-I-79]

<BBC>

Biceps

Brachialis

Coracobrachialis.

All are supplied by musculocutaneous nerve (C5, C6, C7).

8. Elbow: Muscles that Flex it [BCD-I-79]

<Three **B**'s **B**end the elbow>

Biceps

Brachialis

Brachioradialis

☑ Always remember:

- Coracobrachialis is flexor of the arm, not the elbow.
- Brachioradialis is the flexor of elbow, not the arm.
- Brachialis is supplied by both musculocutaneous and radial nerves.

9. Supination and Pronation of Forearm

To **Sup**inate is as if to carry a bowl of **Soup**.

To **Pronate** is as if to **Donate**.

10. Nerve Supply of Serratus Anterior Muscle

Sing in Rhythm:
C5-6-7—Raise your arms to Heaven

Long thoracic nerve supplies the Serratus anterior. Root value of Long thoracic nerve is $C_{5\text{-}6\text{-}7}$ and Serratus anterior helps to raise the arm above 90 degrees.

11. Axillary Artery Branches [BDC-I-48]

<**S**ome **T**imes **L**ife **S**eems **A** **P**ain>
Superior thoracic
Thoracoacromial
Lateral thoracic
Subscapular
Anterior circumflex humeral
Posterior circumflex humeral.

Alternatively: < **S**crew **T**he **L**awyer **S**ave **A** **P**atient >

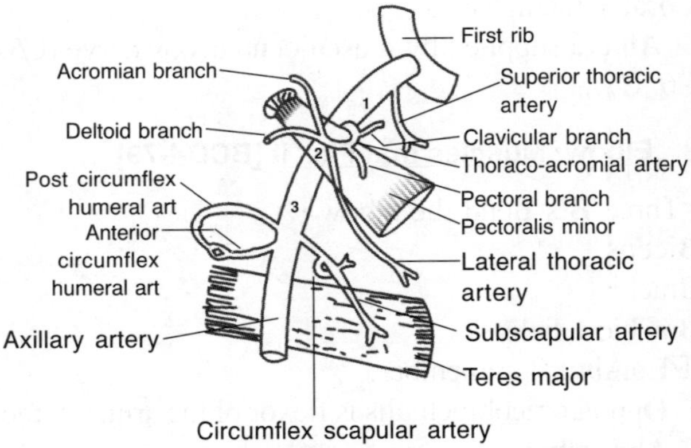

Key: 1–First part, 2–Second part, 3–Third part

Fig.1.5: Axillary artery and its branches

12. Thoracoacromial Artery Branches [BDC-I –48]

<ABCD>
Acromial
Breast (pectoral)
Clavicular
Deltoid.

13. Brachial Artery: Recurrent and Collateral Branches [BDC-I – 84, Fig. 8.9]

<**I** Am **P**retty **S**mart>
Anterior ulnar recurrent artery goes with **I**nferior ulnar collateral artery.
Posterior ulnar recurrent artery goes with **S**uperior ulnar collateral artery.

14. Flexor Muscles of the Forearm [AKD–71]

Superficial group:
<**C**lass **R**epresentatives **C**an **U**sually **P**ersuade **T**eachers to **P**ass **L**ong and **D**ifficult **S**ubjects>
1. flexor **C**arpi **R**adialis
2. flexor **C**arpi **U**lnaris
3. **P**ronator **T**eres
4. **P**lamaris **L**ongus
5. flexor **D**igitorum **S**uperficialis*

* (often described as intermediate layer).

Deep group:
<**P**hysicians and **Q**uacks **P**robably **L**ove **D**oing **PR**>
1. **P**ronator **Q**uadratus
2. flexor **P**olicis **L**ongus
3. flexor **D**igitorum **P**rofundus.

15. Hand Muscles Innervated by Median Nerve [BDC-I -118]

<The **LOAF** muscles>
Lumbricals 1 and 2
Opponens pollicis
Abductor pollicis brevis
Flexor pollicis brevis (superficial head)
Imagine a labourer eating a loaf of bread.
Median nerve is also called the Labourer's nerve
(Alternatively: LLOAF, with 2 L's, to recall there's 2 lumbricals.)

16. Intrinsic Muscles of Hand (Palmar Surface) [BDC-I-108]

<**A**ll **F**or **O**ne **A**nd **O**ne **F**or **A**ll>

Thenar, lateral to medial:
Abductor pollicis brevis
Flexor pollicis brevis
Opponens pollicis
Adductor pollicis.
Hypothenar, lateral to medial:
Opponens digiti minimi
Flexor digiti minimi
Abductor digiti minimi.

17. Interossei Muscles: Actions of Dorsal vs. Palmar in Hand [BDC-I -112]

<PAD and DAB>
The **P**almar **Ad**duct and the **D**orsal **Ab**duct.
Use your hand to dab with a pad.

18. Lumbricals Action [BDC-I -111]

Lumbrical action is to **hold a pea**, that is to flex the metacarpophalangeal joint and extend the interphalangeal joints. When look at hand in this position, can see this makes an **"L"** shape, since L is for Lumbrical.

19. Radial Side in the Wrist

<Mobile users **DIAL** with their **THUMB**>
So the raDIAL side is the side with the THUMB.

20. Carpal Bones [BDC-I -21]

<**S**he **L**ooks **T**oo **P**retty, **T**ry **T**o **C**atch **H**er>
1. **S**caphoid
2. **L**unate
3. **T**riquetrel
4. **P**isiform (smallest)
5. **T**rapezium
6. **T**rapezoid
7. **C**apitate
8. **H**amate.

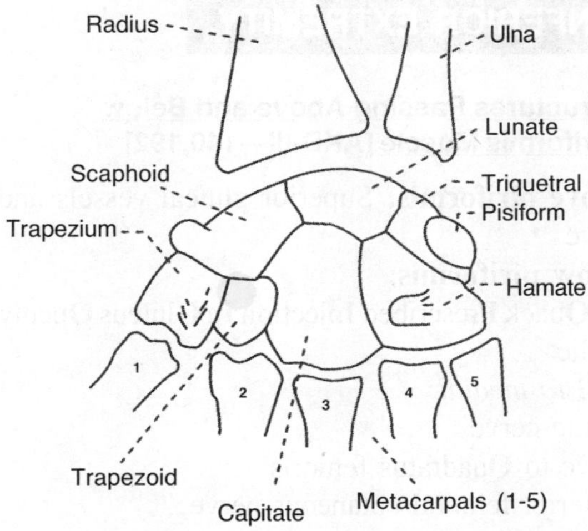

Fig.1.6: Carpal bones in hand

21. <u>Carpal Bones: Trapezium vs. Trapezoid Location</u> [BDC-I -22]

<Trapezi**UM** is by the th**UMB**, Trapez**OID** by its **SIDE**>

22. <u>Structures Passing through Carpal Tunnel</u> [Snell 7th– 520]

<**4 Men** can Fully **Dig Superficial** and **Deep PoLo** Tunnels>
4—4 structures:
Men—Median **n**erve
Fully **Dig Superficial and Deep—F**lexor **Dig**itorum **Superficialis** and **Profundus (deep)**
PoLo—Flexor **Po**licis **Lo**ngus
tunnels—Carpal tunnel.

II. INFERIOR EXTREMITY

1. Structures Passing Above and Below Piriformis Muscle [AKD-III—140,192]

- **Above piriformis:** Superior gluteal vessels and nerve
- **Below piriformis:**

<**S**illy **Q**uack **P**rescribed **I**njection **I**n **G**luteus **O**penly **In** **P**ublic>

Lateral to medial:

1. **S**ciatic nerve
2. Nerve to **Q**uadratus femoris
3. **P**osterior femoral cutaneous nerve
4. **I**nferior **G**luteal nerve
5. **I**nferior **G**luteal vessels
6. Nerve to **O**bturator internus
7. **In**ternal pudendal vessels
8. **P**udendal nerve.

☑ The 3 medial structures appear through the greater sciatic foramen and disappear through lesser sciatic foramen.

2. Inguinal Lymph Nodes [AKD-169]

a. *Superficial group:* (superficial to Fascia Lata) These drain all **superficial structures** below the umbilicus except glans penis.

a. Subcutaneous structures of anterior abdominal wall below the umbilicus
b. Penis including the prepuce
c. Scrotum
d. Vulva
e. Vagina below the hymen*
f. Lower part of anal canal below the pectinate line*
g. Perineum
h. Gluteal region
i. Afferents from the superficial lymph nodes of lower limb

(*Considering them superficial as these are derivatives of the ectoderm)

b. *Deep Inguinal group:* (Deep to Fascia Lata)

<Glans goes deepest inside, and it's very spongy there!>

These drain:

a. Glans penis

b. Spongy (penile) part of male urethra.

☑ They are 1-3 in number.

☑ Gland of **Cloquet** is present in femoral canal.

Note:

- The testes do not drain in inguinal lymph nodes.
- Efferent lymphatics from superficial and deep inguinal lymph nodes drain into external iliac nodes.

3. Femoral Triangle: Floor

<**I**diot **P**une **M**ust **P**olish **A**ll **F**loors>

<**I**ndian **P**rime **M**inister **P**aid **A**ll **F**armers>

I—Iliacus

PM—Psoas Major

P—Pectineus

A—Adductor longus

Floor—Floor of femoral triangle

☑ **A**dductor magnus is included in **A**natomical femoral triangle.

☑ (Femoral triangle without Adductor Magnus is called Geometric Triangle)

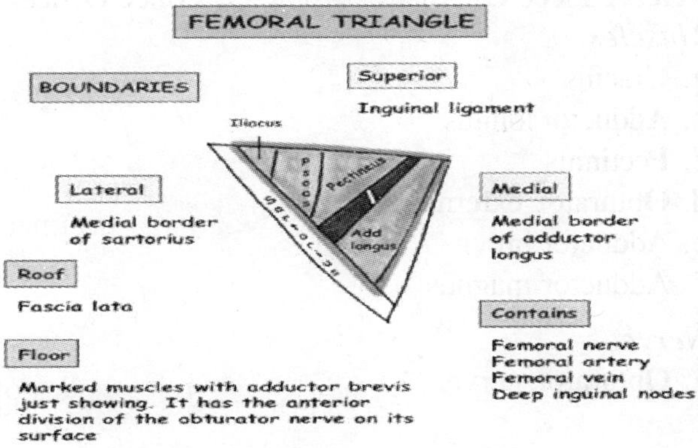

Fig.1.7: Carpal bones in hand

4. Contents of Femoral Triangle [AKD-III-173] [BDC-II-43]

<Femoral—**FLAG VAN**>
1. **F**ibrofatty tissue
2. **L**ymph nodes (Deep inguinal)
3. **A** part of lateral femoral cutaneous nerve
4. **G**enito-femoral nerve
5. Femoral **V**ein
6. Femoral **A**rtery
7. Femoral **N**erve.

5. Coverings of Complete Femoral Hernia [AKD-178]

<**S**ome **S**chools **C**ancelled **A**dmission of **F**ools **P**ermanently>

Superficial to deep:

a. **S**kin
b. **S**uperficial fascia
c. **C**ribriform fascia
d. **A**nterior wall of femoral sheath
e. **F**emoral septum
f. **P**eritoneum of hernial sac

☑ **P**rofunda **F**emoris artery has **F**our **P**reforators.

6. Contents of Adductor Compartment [AKD-184]

<**G**et **A** **P**iece **O**f **A**dam's **A**pple **O**f **P**olice **O**fficer>

Muscles:

a. **G**racilis
b. **A**dductor longus
c. **P**ectinius
d. **O**bturator externus
e. **A**dductor brevis
f. **A**dductor magnus

Nerve:

a. **O**bturator nerve.

Arteries:

a. **P**rofunda femoris artery.

b. **O**bturator artery.

7. Insertion Of Ilio-Psoas tendon:

<My **Sore Ass** was a **Little Tortured** >

Here's a way to remember the insertion of the iliopsoas common tendon:

It inserts on the lesser trochanter of the femur. So, you remember it by thinking that if you have a sore ass (so' ass —psoas), you want to sit less.

8. Hamstring Muscles: [AKD-199]

<BLISS>

BL – **B**iceps femoris-**L**ong head

I – **I**schial fibers of Adductor Magnus

S – **S**emimembranosus

S – **S**emitendinosus

- ☑ Only Semimembranosus and Semitendinosus are true hamstrings.
- ☑ Oblique popliteal ligament is a continuation of semimembranosus.

9. Hamstring Muscles: Criteria [AKD-199]

<FITS>

F- **F**lexors of knee & extensors of hip joint

I- **I**schial tuberosity origin

T- **T**ibia or fibula insertion

S- **S**ciatic nerve supply

10. Contents of Popliteal fossa: [AKD-204]

<**P**ublic **T**oilets **C**an **S**ometimes **G**ive **A** **L**ittle **P**rivacy>

1. **P**opliteal artery & vein
2. **T**ibial nerve
3. **C**ommon peroneal nerve
4. **S**mall saphenous vein
5. **G**enicular branch of posterior division of obturator nerve
6. **A** pad of fat

7. **L**ymph nodes
8. **P**osterior femoral cutaneous nerve

11. Contents of Flexor Compartment of Leg: [AKD-209]

<Some **G**ood **P**atients **P**ay **F**ull **F**ees **T**o **N**ew **P**hysicians>

Superficial part:
1. **S**oleus
2. **G**astrocnemius
3. **P**lantaris

Deep part:

4. **P**oplitius
5. **F**lexor hallucis longus
6. **F**lexor digitorum longus
7. **T**ibialis posterior
8. **N**erve (Tibial nerve)
9. **P**osterior tibial and peroneal vessels

12. Inversion vs. Eversion Muscles in Leg [BDC-II – 83,90,99]

<Second letter rule for inversion/eversion >

Eversion muscles:

p**E**rineus longus

p**E**rineus brevis

p**E**rineus tertius

Inversion muscles:

t**I**bialis anterior

t**I**bialis posterior

13. Soleus vs. Gastrocnemius Muscle Function [BDC-II – 96]

<Stand on your Soles. Explosive Gas>

You stand on soles of your shoes, so Soleus is for posture.

Gasoline is explosive, so Gastrocnemius is for explosive movement.

14. Tarsal Bones

<**C**hacha **C**haudhuri **L**oves **MINT**>

1. **C**alcaneus
2. **C**uboid
3. **L**ateral cuneiform
4. **M**edial cuneiform
5. **I**ntermediate cuneiform
6. **N**avicular
7. **T**alus

15. Tibia vs. Fibula

Can't tell your tibia from your fibula?
The **T**ibia is the **T**hick, inner **B**one. The **Fibula** is **F**iner, **F**luted, and **L**ateral.

16. Buttock Quadrant Safest for Needle Insertion [BDC-II –64]

<Shut **U**p and butt **O**ut>
(Imagine a nurse with injection in hand telling a patient to shut up & show his butt.)
The **Upper Outer** quadrant of the Buttock safely avoids hitting sciatic nerve.

17. Inguinal Canal: Walls [BDC-II -177]

<MALT: 2M, 2A, 2L, 2T>
Starting from superior, moving around in order to posterior:
Superior wall (roof): **2 Muscles:**
-internal oblique **M**uscle
-transversus abdominis **M**uscle
Anterior wall: **2 Aponeuroses:**
Aponeurosis of external oblique
Aponeurosis of internal oblique
Lower wall (floor): **2 Ligaments:**
inguinal **L**igament
lacunar **L**igament
Posterior wall: **2Ts:**
fascia **T**ransversalis
conjoint **T**endon

18. Medial Malleolus: Order of Tendons, Artery, Nerve Behind it [BDC-II-21]

<**T**om**,** **D**ick **AN** **H**arry>

From anterior to posterior:

1. **T**ibialis Posterior
2. **D**igitorum
3. **A**rtery
4. **N**erve
5. **H**allucis

Full names for these are: Tibialis Posterior, Flexor Digitorum Longus, Posterior Tibial Artery, Posterior Tibial Nerve, and Flexor Hallucis Longus.

☑ Alternatively: (*in hindi*) <**T**ulsi **D**as **A**mir **N**ahi **H**ai>

19. The Muscles Attached to Tibia's Medial Side [BDC-II –21, 22]

<A **Girl** between 2 **Sargeants**>
Gracilus is between
Sartorius and
Semitendonosus

20. Cruciate Ligaments of Knee Joint: [AKD-247] [BDC-127]

- **A**nterior cruciate ligament is attached **A**nteriorly on the tibia and prevents **A**nterior displacement of tibia.
- **P**osterior cruciate ligament is attached **P**osteriorly on the tibia and prevents **P**osterior displacement of tibia.

21. Attachments to Intercondylar Area of Tibia: [AKD-242]

Anterior to posterior:
<Medial Condyle Looks Like Medial Condyle!>

1. Anterior horn of **M**edial meniscus
2. Anterior **C**ruciate ligament
3. Anterior horn of **L**ateral meniscus

4. Posterior horn of **L**ateral meniscus
5. Posterior horn of **M**edial meniscus
6. Posterior **C**ruciate ligament

☑ Alternatively: <**M**edical **C**ollege **L**ahore **L**acks **M**edicine **C**abinets>

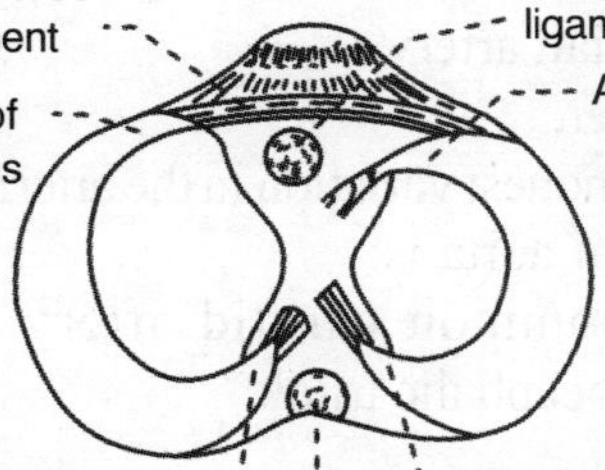

Fig. 1.6: Upper articular surface of right Tibia and the structures attached to the intercondylar area

22. Subcutaneous Bursa Around the Knee Joint: [AKD-251]

<House maids **Pre**pare **P**lates>
House Maid's bursa is **Pre-P**atellar bursa.
Sometimes this bursa is swollen in house maids due to washing of floor in kneel down position.

<Clergyman **In** **P**rayer>
Clergyman's bursa is **In**fra **P**atellar bursa.
This bursa is sometimes swollen in persons during prayer in kneel down position with trunk upright.

III. THORAX

1. Aortic Arch Branches [Gray 38th-1513]

"Know your ABC'S"

Aortic arch gives…
Bracheiocephalic trunk
left **C**ommon Carotid
left **S**ubclavian artery.

☑ Remember:

The commonest variation in the arteries arising form the arch of aorta is:

- Left common carotid artery arising from brachiocephalic trunk.

2. Diaphragm Apertures: Spinal Levels [BDC-I–161] [AKD-177]

Aortic hiatus = 12 letters = T12
Oesophagus = 10 letters = T10
Vena cava = 8 letters = T8.

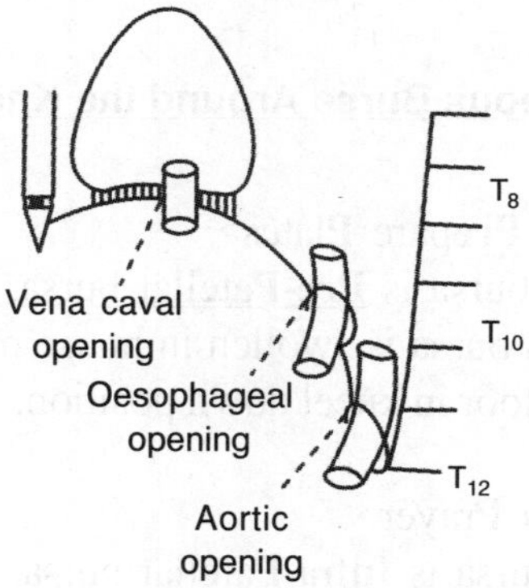

Fig. 1.7: Major openings in the Diaphragm

3. Diaphragm Innervation [AKD-117]

<3, 4, 5 keeps the diaphragm alive>

The motor supply of the diaphragm is solely from the phrenic nerve (C_3, C_4, and C_5).

4. Superior Mediastinum: Contents [BDC-I–210]

<PVT. Left BATTLE>

1. **P**hrenic nerve
2. **V**agus nerve
3. **T**horacic duct
4. **Le**ft recurrent laryngeal nerve (not the right)
5. **B**rachiocephalic veins
6. **A**ortic arch (and its 3 branches)
7. **T**hymus
8. **T**rachea
9. **L**ymph nodes
10. **E**sophagus

5. Posterior Mediastinum Structures [BDC-I –212]

There are 4 birds **<3 goose and a duck>**
The esophaGOOSE (esophagus)
The vaGOOSE nerve (vagus)
The azyGOOSE vein (azygos, hemiazygos and accessory hemiazygos)
The thoracic DUCK (duct)
(***Also descending thoracic aorta).

6. Thoracic Duct: Relation to Azygous Vein and Esophagus [BDC-I–212]

<The duck between 2 gooses>
Thoracic duct (duck) is between 2 gooses, azygos and esophagus.

7. Vagus Nerve: Path into Thorax

<my **A**unt **Left V**egas in **T**hrash>
Left Vagus nerve goes **A**nterior descending into the **T**horax.

8. Bronchopulmonary Segments of Right Lung [BDC-I –206]

<**A PALM S**eed **M**akes **A**nother **L**ittle **P**alm>
In order from superior to inferior:
Upper lobe:

1. **A**pical

2. **P**osterior
3. **A**nterior

Middle lobe:

4. **L**ateral
5. **M**edial

Lower lobe:

6. **S**uperior (Apical)
7. **M**edial basal
8. **A**nterior basal
9. **L**ateral basal
10. **P**osterior basal.

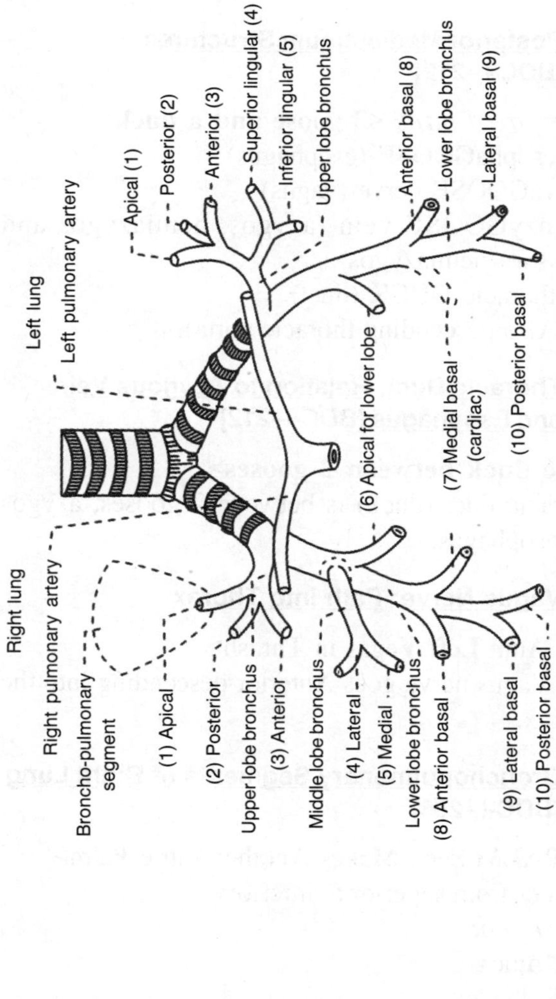

Fig.1.8: Distribution of tertiary bronchi in right and left lungs

9. <u>Pleura</u>: <u>Surface Markings</u> [BDC-I–197, 203]

<All the even ribs, in order: 2, 4, 6, 8, 10, 12 show its route>

Rib 2: Runs straight down from here

Rib 4: The left pleura does a lateral shift to accommodate heart

Rib 6: Both diverge laterally.

Rib 8: Midclavicular line

Rib 10: Midaxillary line

Rib 12: The back (lateral border of sacrospinalis muscle).

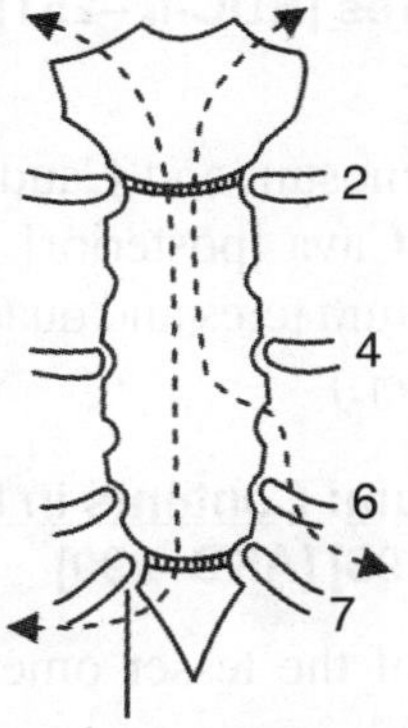

Fig. 1.9: Costo-mediastinal reflexion of pleurae

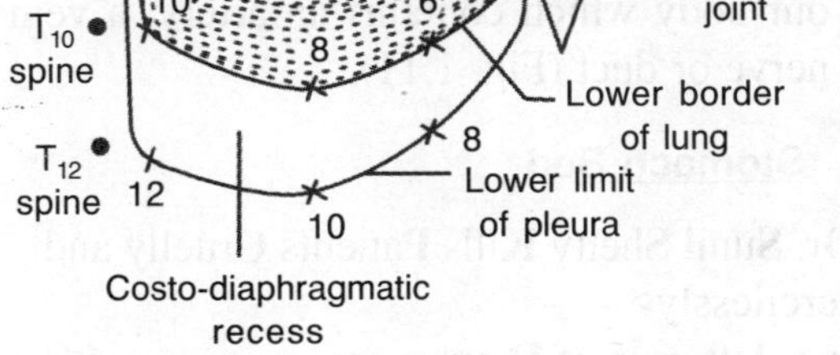

Fig. 1.10: Costo-diaphragmatic recess (Right lateral view)

10. **P**arietal pleura and **P**arietal peritoneum are **P**ain sensitive.

IV. ABDOMEN

1. Duodenum: Lengths of Parts [BDC-II–213]

<Counting 1 to 4 but staggered >
1st part: 2 inches
2nd part: 3 inches
3rd part: 4 inches
4th part: 1 inch
☑ Total = 10 inches or 25 cm
☑ 1 inch = 2.5 cm

2. Liver: Side with ligamentum venosum/ caudate lobe vs. side with quadrate lobe/ ligamentum teres [BDC-II –251]

< **VC** goes with **VC** >
The ligamentum **V**enosum and **C**audate lobe are on same side as **V**ena **C**ava [posterior].
(Therefore, ligamentum teres and quadrate lobe must be on anterior of liver.)

3. Lesser Omentum: Contents in Right Free Margin [BDC -195] [AKD -290]

Right free margin of the lesser omentum (epiploic foramen) contains:
Anterior to posterior: **<BHP>**
Bile duct
Hepatic artery
Portal vein
☑ Note: It is one of the series of vascular triads in our body which contains an artery, a vein and a nerve or duct (Fig. 1.11).

4. Stomach Bed

<**Dr.** **S**unil **S**hetty **K**ills **P**atients **C**ruelly and **M**ercilessly>
Dr. = left crus of **D**iaphragm
Sunil = **S**plenic artery
Shetty = left **S**uprarenal gland
Kills = left **K**idney
Patients = body of **P**ancreas

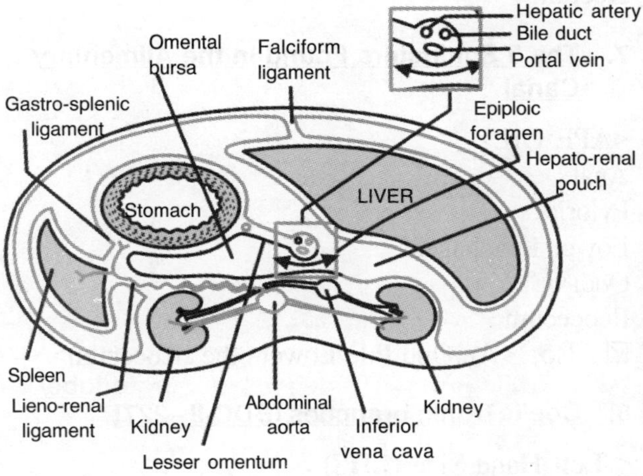

Fig. 1.11: Transverse section through the epiploic foramen

Cruelly = left **C**olic flexure
Mercilessly = transverse **M**esocolon
☑ Remember the stomach lies over the Lesser Omentum.

5. Parts of the Stomach

<Driving **CAR** is **FUN** till the **BODIES PILE** up>
CARDIA
FUNdus
BODY
PYLorus.

6. Bowel Segments

<**D**ow **J**ones **I**ndustrial **A**verages **C**losing **S**tock **R**eport >
Duodenum
Jejunum
Ileum
Appedix
Cecum / **C**olon

Sigmoid
Rectum

7. The 5 Sphincters Found in the Alimentary Canal

<APE OIL>
Anal
Pyloric
Lower Esophageal
Oddi
Ileocecum
☑ Also, <An Odd Pile Lowers the Ileocecum>

8. Coelic trunk: branches [BDC-II –227]

< **L**eft **H**and **S**ide **(LHS)** >
Left gastric artery
Hepatic artery (common hepatic)
Splenic artery

9. Abdominal Aorta Branches: [BDC-II –272]

<**P**rostitutes **C**ause **S**agging **S**wollen **R**ed **T**esticles (in men) **L**iving **I**n **S**in >
1. **P**hrenic [inferior]
2. **C**eliac
3. **S**uperior mesenteric
4. **S**uprarenal [middle]
5. **R**enal
6. **T**esticular [**"in men"** only]
7. **L**umbars
8. **I**nferior mesenteric
9. **S**acral

10. Inferior Vena Cava Tributaries [BDC-II –272]

<**I** **L**ike **T**o **R**ise **S**o **H**igh>
a. **I**lliacs
b. **L**umbar
c. **T**esticular
d. **R**enal
e. **S**uprarenal

f. **H**epatic vein.

Think of the IVC wanting to rise high up to the heart.

11. Internal Iliac Artery: Branches [BDC-II –340]

From Anterior division:

<**S**ome **O**bstruction **I**n **M**y **I**nternal **I**liac>

1. **S**uperior vesical artery. (Obliterated umbilical A.)
2. **O**bturator
3. **I**nferior vesical
4. **M**iddle rectal
5. **I**nternal pudendal
6. **I**nferior gluteal

From posterior division

<**I** **L**ike **S**exy **G**irls>

7. **I**liolumbar
8. **L**ateral sacral
9. **S**uperior **G**luteal

12. Meckel's Diverticulum Details [R-830]

<Rule of 2>

2 inches long

2 feet proximal to ileocecal valve

2 times more common in men

2% occurrence in population

2 types of tissues may be present (gastric & pancreatic)

☑ Remember: **"di-"** means **"two"**, so diverticulum is the thing with all the twos.

13. Ureter to Ovarian/Testicular Artery Relation [BDC-II –262]

<Water under the bridge>

The ureters (which carry water), are posterior to the ovarian/testicular artery.

Clinically important, since a common surgical error is to cut ureter instead of ovarian artery when removing uterus.

14. Spleen: Dimensions, Weight, Surface Anatomy [BDC-II –243]

<Odd Numbers: 1,3,5,7,9,11>
Spleen dimensions are 1 inch x 3 inches x 5 inches.
Weight is 7 ounces (1 ounce is approx. 30gms)
It lies under the ribs 9 to 11.

15. Oblique Muscles of Abdomen: Direction of Externals vs. Internals [BDC-II –168]

<Hands in your pockets >
When put hands in your pockets, fingers now lie on top of external obliques and fingers point their direction of fibers: down and towards midline.
Note: **"oblique"** tells that must be going at an angle.
☑ Internal obliques are at right angles to external.

16. Lumbar plexus [BDC-II –38]

<**I**nterested **I**n **G**etting **L**aid **O**n **F**ridays?>
1. **I**liohypogastric [L1]
2. **I**lioinguinal [L1]
3. **G**enitofemoral [L1, L2]
4. **L**ateral femoral cutaneous [L2, L3]
5. **O**bturator [L2, L3, L4]
6. **F**emoral [L2, L3, L4]

17. Lumbar plexus roots

<2 from 1, 2 from 2, 2 from 3>
2 nerves from 1 root: Ilioinguinal (L1), Iliohypogastric (L1).
2 nerves from 2 roots: Genitofemoral (L1,L2), Lateral Femoral (L2,L3).
2 nerves from 3 roots: Obturator (L2,L3,L4), Femoral (L2,L3,L4).

18. Cremastric reflex: [BDC-II-172] [Snell-5th-149]

The cremastic muscles can be made to contract by stroking the skin on the medial aspect of the thigh, known as the cremastric reflex.

Nerve supply is through the **Genitofemoral** nerve (L1 , L2)

It's quite easy to remember the afferent and efferent:

Think of the thigh and femur comes to the mind … so the afferent is Femoral branch of genitofemoral nerve.

Think of the cremaster and the genitals come to the mind … so the efferent is the Genital branch of genitofemoral nerve.

Boys have 1 penis and 2 testes … so the root value is L1, L2.

Also associate the chromosome location for gene of testicular carcinoma …which is 12.

19. Penis Autonomic Innervation Actions [BDC-II –307]

<Point and Shoot>

Parasympathetic **P**oints the **P**enis, **S**ympathetic **S**hoots out the **S**emen.

(Erection and Ejaculation)

<**P**arasympathetic causes **P**otty & **P**ee>

Parasympathetic causes defecation & urination

***Note: Parasympathetic – S2,S3,S4
Sympathetic (T11 to L2)

20. Innervation of the penis

<S2,3,4 keeps the penis off the floor>

The parasympathetic innervation of the penis is by the pudendal nerve which is derived from spinal cord levels S2, S3, S4.

Alternatively:

<S2,3,4 keeps the 3 P's off the floor (Potty, Pee & Penis)>

☑ S2,3,4 causes:

- Constriction of anal sphincter
- Constriction of Urethral sphincter, and
- Erection of penis

21. Splanchnic Nerves:

<Splanchnic nerves = medical students >
Study from 9-5,
Take a break between 10-11
Go home at 12.

Greater splanchnic = T5-T9
Lesser splanchnic = T10-T11
Least splanchnic = T12

☑ Also Remember
Pelvic splanchic = **P**arasympathetic
Sacral splanchic = **S**ympathetic

22. Dematomes on Abdomen

T10 is at the belly **butTEN** (**button**)
L1 is at the **I**nguinal **L**igament.(**IL**=**L1**)

23. Scrotum layers [BDC-II –184]

<**S**ome **D**amn **E**nglishman **C**alled **I**t **T**he **T**estis>
From superficial to deep:
1. **S**kin
2. **D**artos
3. **E**xternal spermatic fascia
4. **C**remaster
5. **I**nternal spermatic fascia
6. **T**unica vaginalis
7. **T**estis

24. Sperm Pathway Through Male Reproductive Tract [Ganong-428]

<SEVEN UP>
1. **S**eminiferous tubules
2. **E**pididymis
3. **V**as deferens
4. **E**jaculatory duct
5. (**N**othing)
6. **U**rethra
7. **P**enis

25. Spermatic Cord Contents [BDC-II –179]

<**P**iles **D**on't **C**ontribute **T**o **A** **G**ood **S**ex **L**ife>

1. **P**ampiniform plexus
2. **D**uctus deferens
3. **C**remasteric artery
4. **T**esticular artery
5. **A**rtery of the ductus deferens
6. **G**enital branch of the genitofemoral nerve
7. **S**ympathetic nerve fibers
8. **L**ymphatic vessels

Another good one :

26. Spermatic Cord Contents

<**CAT** **G**ut **L**igature **P**rovides **Vas**t **P**rotection>

- **C**remastric **A**nd **T**esticular artery
- **G**enital Branch of genitofemoral nerve
- **L**ymphatics
- **P**rocessus Vaginalis (its remains)
- **Vas** deferens
- **P**ampiniform plexus

27. Mesonephric and Paramesonephric Duct [I.B.Singh 274, 290]

Mesonephric duct = Wolffian duct
Paramesonephric duct = Mullerian duct
Mnemonic: <The shorter name goes with the shorter name and longer with longer>

Wolffian duct gives rise to males (Wolf = male)
Mullerian duct gives rise to females (Mother = females)

28. Common Structures Made by Wolffian Duct in Male and Female

<**CoCa** (cola), **Pe**psi & **T**humbs **U**p **Po**ssibly **W**ent in **urine**>

- **Co**llecting tubules
- **Ca**lyces
- **Pe**lvis

- **T**rigone of bladder
- **U**reters
- **Po**sterior part of urethra
- **W**olffian duct
- **Urine** – helps you to remember that all these are parts of urinary tract.

29. Wolffian Duct Derived Structures in Males and Females

In males:

<Male has **A SEED**>

A—Appendix of epididymis
S—**S**eminal vesical
E—**E**pididymis
E—**E**jaculatory duct
D—**D**uctus deferens

In females:

<PEG>

Paraophoron
Epoophoron (organ of Rosenmuller)
Gartner's duct

30. Mullerian Duct: Special Structures in Females

<FUCx **U>**

Fallopian tubes
Uterus
Cervix
Upper ¾ of vagina

☑ *In males*: It forms **appendix of testis**.

31. Appendix of Testis and Appendix of Epididymis : Origin [I.B.Singh – 278, 291]

<**PT** **M**orning & **E**vening>

P=T : **P**aramesonephric duct gives *appendix of Testis*
M=E : **M**esonephric duct gives *appendix of Epididymis*

32. Hormones Secreted by Sartoli Cells

<Sartoli has an AIM>
Androgen binding protein
Inhibin
Mullerian inhibiting substance

Other functions of sartoli cells:
< 4P's >
Provide nutrition to developing sperm cells
Phagocytoze injured or dead sperm cells
Prevents substances from entering the lumen of seminiferous tubules (Blood testis barrier)
Produce some estrogen from testosterone.

33. Sartoli vs. Leydig Cells: [SKC-243]

- **Sartoli** cells: come to **Sort** out the sex confusion (secretes mullerian inhibiting substance) and it is present only in **Sirs** (males).
- **Leydig cells** : "You need real **Testosterone** to *lay* and *dig* her" . Leydig cells secrete testosterone.

34. Broad Ligament: Contents [BDC-II –318,322]

<BROAD ligament>
a. **B**undle (ovarian neurovascular bundle)
b. **R**ound ligament
c. **O**varian ligament
d. **A**dditional vestigial structures (Eoophoron, paraoophoron, Gartner duct)
e. **D**uct (oviduct)

35. Muscles Attached to Perineal Body : [BDC-II-285, Fig.-28.4]

<BLESSeD>
a. **B**ulbospongiosus
b. **L**evator ani
c. **E**xternal anal sphincter muscles
d. **S**phincter urethrae
e. **S**uperficial transverse perini
f. **D**eep transverse perini

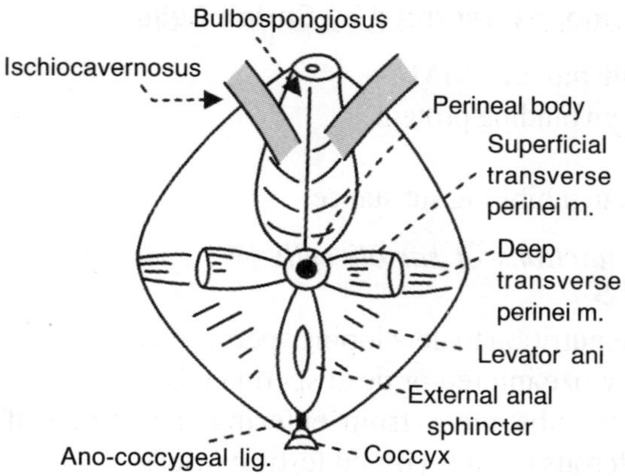

Fig. 1.12: The perineal body and the anococcygeal ligament

36. Pelvic Diaphragm — -Posterior to anterior

<**H**ot **COLA**>
Piriformis (**'pyro'** means hot)
COccygeus,
Levator **A**ni

37. Kidney Hilum at Transpyloric Plane (L1) [BDC-II-257]

<**L-1** goes through hilum of only **1** kidney, and it's the **L**eft one>

38. Left Renal Vein: Tributaries [Gray's -38th-1601]

<**GPS**>
- Left **G**onadal
- Left inferior **P**hrenic
- Left **S**uprarenal

39. Umbilical Cord [Ref. Dutta 4th/40]

1. Initially has two veins and two arteries
2. By 4th month of intrauterine life à Right vein disappears. So, now umbilical cord has:
   i. Right and left Arteries
   ii. Left vein.

[Mnemonic: "Right died in the **fight; Left vein** is left in **pain"]**

- *Fully developed umbilical cord is on* average 50 cm *long and 1-2 cm in diameter (range of length 20-120 cm).*
- *Valves of* **HOBOKEN** *are present in umbilical vessels particularly artery (Ref.* Gray 37th-143).
  Ref. Langeman's 8th/244
- *After birth the proximal portions of the umbilical arteries persists as the Internal iliac and superior vesical arteries and distal parts are obliterated to form the medial umbilical ligaments.*
  Ref. Langeman's 8th/248
- After birth the *left umbilical vein* and *ductus venosus* are obliterated and form the *ligamentum teres hepatis and ligamentum venosum* respectively.
  Ref. Dutta 4th/40
- Presence of a single umbilical artery is often associated with fetal congenital abnormalities.

V.. HEAD AND NECK

1. Bell's Palsy: Symptoms

<BELL'S Palsy>
Blink reflex abnormal
Earache
Lacrimation [deficient, excess]
Loss of taste
Sudden onset
Palsy of VII nerve muscles
(All symptoms are unilateral).

2. Pterygoid Muscles: Lateral vs. Medial [BDC-III-117]

<Look at how your jaw ends up when saying first syllable of 'Lateral' or 'Medial'>
"La": Your jaw is now open, so lateral opens mouth.
"Me": Your jaw is still closed, so medial closes the mandible.

3. Internal Jugular Vein: Tributaries [BDC-III-149]

<**M**edical **S**chools **L**et **C**onfident **P**eople **I**n>:
From inferior to superior:
Middle thyroid
Superior thyroid
Lingual
Common facial
Pharyngeal
Inferior petrosal sinus.

4. Maxillary Artery: Branches [BDC-III-119]

<DAMIAn chew PIG AS PAM>
First Part:
- **D**eep auricular
- **A**nterior tympanic
- **M**iddle meningeal
- **I**nferior alveolar
- **A**ccessory meningeal (Nothing).

Second Part: **(Muscles that chew+buccal)**

Masseteric
Pterygoid
Deep temporal
Buccal

Third Part:

Pharyngeal
Infraorbital
Greater palatine
Artery of the pterygoid canal
Sphenopalatine
Posterior superior alveolar
Anterior superior alveolar
Middle superior alveolar

5. Portal-Systemic Anastomoses: Main Two Places that Retroperitoneals Connect into Systemic

<**R**etro**P**eritoneals hook up with **R**enal and **P**aravertebral veins>

6. <u>Scalp Layers</u> [BDC-III-37]

"SCALP"

(From superficial to deep)

1. **S**kin
2. **C**onnective tissue
3. **A**poneurosis
4. **L**oose areolar tissue
5. **P**ericranium.

7. <u>Trigeminal nerve: where branches exit skull [BDC-III-24]</u>

<**O**h! **M**y **M**an has **S**tanding **R**oom **O**nly>

Oh—Opthalmic nv.
My – Maxillary nv.
Man – Mandibular nv.
Standing — **Superior** orbital fissure is V1 (Opthalmic nv.)
Room — foramen **Rotundum** is V2 (Maxillary nv.)
Only — foramen **Ovale** is V3 (Mandibular nv.)

8. V3 (Mandibular Nerve) Innervated Muscles [BDC-III-125]

(1st branchial arch derivatives)

< MD My TV >

Mastication [masseter, temporalis, pterygoids]
Digastric [anterior belly]
Mylohyoid
tensor **T**ympani
tensor **V**eli palatini

9. V3: Sensory Branches [BDC-III-125,126]

<**B**uccaneers **A**re **I**nferior **L**inguists>
<BAIL>
Buccal (only sensory branch from anterior trunk)
Auriculo-temporal
Inferior alveolar
Lingual

10. Voice Box: Names of Parts in Sagittal Cross-section

<There's **3 V's** in your Voicebox>
Vestibular fold
Ventricle
Vocal fold
☑ Note: Vestibular and Vocal cord also known as false and true cords respectively.

11. Foramen Ovale Contents [BDC-III-24]

<OVALE>
Otic ganglion lies just below it
V3 cranial nerve (Mandibular)
Accessory meningeal artery
Lesser petrosal nerve
Emissary veins (connecting cavernous sinus with pterygoid plexus of veins)

12. Structures Passing Through Supraorbital Fissure: [BDC-III-25]

<**L**azy **F**rench **T**arts **S**it **N**aked **I**n **A**nticipation **O**f **S**ex>
Lacrimal nerve
Frontal nerve
Trochlear nerve
Superior branch of oculomotor nerve
Nasociliary nerve
Inferior branch of oculomotor nerve
Abducent nerve
Ophthalmic veins (sup. & inf.)
Sympathetic nerves

13. Cavernous Sinus: Structures Passing Through [BDC –III-94]

"Once upon a time **Nerves 3, 4, 5 & 6** went To a **Cave In Car**.
Nerve 5 was so nervous that it **left its 3rd part (V_3) behind in Ovale**.
Once in the cave only **number 6** had the courage to take the **Car** to the **center** of the cave.
Rest of them stayed close to the walls."

Structures in the lateral wall of sinus from above downwards:
a. Occulomotor (**III**[rd]) nerve
b. Trochlear (**IV**[th]) nerve
c. Opthalmic (V_1) nerve
d. Maxillary (V_2) nerve
e. Trigeminal ganglion

Structures passing through center of cavernous sinus
a. Abducent (**VIth**) nerve
b. **In**ternal **Car**otid artery

Cave – **Cave**rnous sinus
In Car – **In**ternal **Car**otrid
*** Mandibular nerve (V3) passes through foramen ovale.

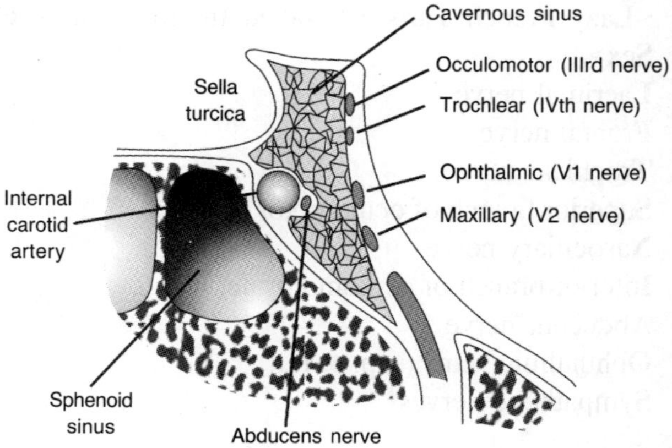

Fig. 1.13

14. True and False Capsule Arrangement in Thyroid and Prostate [BDC-III-136,139]

In **T**hyroid surgery: **T**ake away **T**rue capsule
In **P**rostate surgery: **P**reserve both capsule

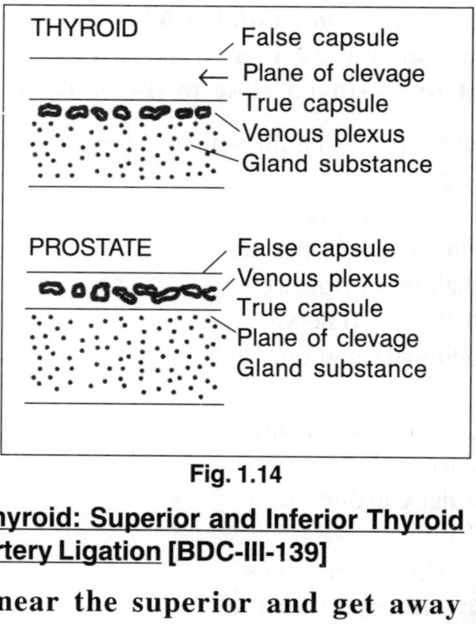

Fig. 1.14

15. Thyroid: Superior and Inferior Thyroid Artery Ligation [BDC-III-139]

"Go near the superior and get away from inferiors"

During operation of the thyroid gland, superior thyroid artery is ligated near the gland to save the external laryngeal nerve; and inferior thyroid artery is ligated away from the gland to save the recurrent laryngeal nerve.

16. Thyroid Artery and Thyroid Vein Relation

"Upper birth for newly married
Middle birth for bachelor
Lower birth for divorced"

- Superior thyroid vein is closely related to Superior thyroid artery.
- Middle thyroid vein does not have corresponding thyroid artery.
- Inferior thyroid vein goes far from inferior thyroid artery.

17. Branches of the Superior Thyroid Artery

"**M**ay **I** **S**ofty **S**queeze **C**ute **G**irls?"
Muscular
Infrahyoid
Superior laryngeal
Sternomastoid
Cricothyroid
Glandular.

18. Meninges [BDC-III-244]

<**PAD**> from within our wards:
Pia mater
Arachnoid mater
Dura mater

19. Communications between Ventricles of Brain and Subarachnoid Space [BDC-III-248]

Foramen of **M**agendie is **M**edian foramen.
Foramen of **L**uschka is **L**ateral foramen.

20. Descending Tracts of Spinal Cord [BDC-III-248]

"**C**elina **R**ubs **O**il **V**ery **T**actfully and **R**elaxes **M**ost **L**ovingly"
Corticospinal tract (Lateral and Anterior)

Rubrospinal tract
Olivospinal tract
Vestibulospinal tract
Tectospinal tract
Retoiculospinal tract (Lateral and Medial)
Medial **L**ongitudinal bundle

☑ Corticospinal tract is also called Pyramidal tract. Lateral tract is crossed and anterior tract is uncrossed.

☑ All descending tracts have '-spinal' as post-fix except medial longitudinal bundle.

21. Ascending Tracts in Spinal Cord [BDC-III-248]

1. Posterior **F**uniculus has 2 **F**asciculus (Posterior column tracts)
   a. **F**asciculus gracilis (medially)
   b. **F**asciculus cuneatus (laterally).
2. Lateral Funiculus has 4 **'Spino-'** tracts
   a. Lateral **Spino**thalamic tract
   b. Anterior and posterior **Spino**cerebellar tract
   c. **Spino**-olivary tract
   d. **Spino**-tectal tract
3. **Anterior** Funiculus has only **Anterior** Spino-thalamic tract (Fig. 1.15).

22. Cranial Nerves

"**O**..**O**..**O**h! **T**o **T**ouch **A**nd **F**eel **A** **G**irl's **V**agina, **AH**!"

1. **O**lfactory
2. **O**ptic
3. **O**cculomotor
4. **T**rochlear
5. **T**rigeminal
6. **A**bducent
7. **F**acial
8. **A**uditory
9. **G**lossopharyngeal
10. **V**agus
11. **A**ccessory
12. **H**ypoglossus

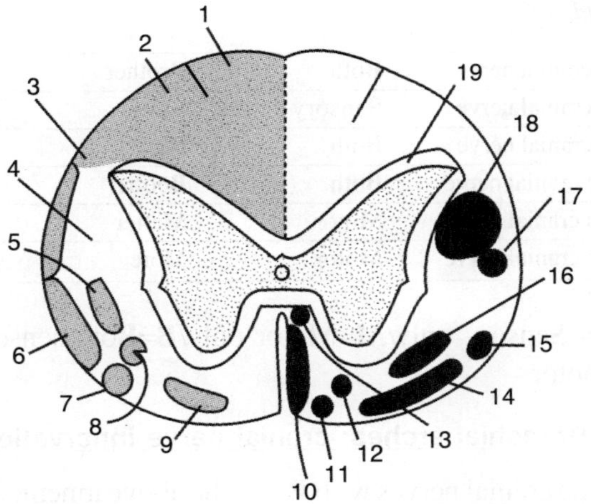

Fig. 1.15: Transverse section of the spinal cord showing the main ascending and descending tracts (1) Fasciculus gracilis (2) Fasciculus cuneatus (3) Dorsolateral tract (4) Posterior spino-cerebellar tract (5) Lateral spino-thalamic tract (6) Ant. spino-cerebellar tract (7) Spino-olivary tract (8) Spinotectal tract (9) Ant. spinothalamic tract (10) Anterior corticospinal tract (11) Tectospinal tract (12) Medial reticulospinal tract (13) Medial longitudinal bundle (14) Vestibulospinal tract (15) Olivospinal tract (16) Lateral reticulo-spinal tract (17) Rubrospinal tract (18) Lateral corticospinal tract (19) Intersegmental tracts

☑ **You have one nose. You have two eyes, so the first "O" is Olfactory; second "O" is Optic.**

☑ **3,4,6 makes my eyes do Tricks . (These three nerves supply the extra ocular muscles)**

23. Cranial Nerves: Sensory, Motor or Both

<**S**ome **S**ay **M**arry **M**oney **B**ut **M**y **B**rother **S**ays **B**ig **B**oobs **M**atter **M**ore>

1st cranial nerve	**S**ensory	**S**ome
2nd cranial nerve	**S**ensory	**S**ay
3rd cranial nerve	**M**otor	**M**arry
4th cranial nerve	**M**otor	**M**oney
5th cranial nerve	**B**oth	**B**ut
6th cranial nerve	**M**otor	**M**y

Contd.

Contd.

7th cranial nerve	**B**oth	**B**rother
8th cranial nerve	**S**ensory	**S**ays
9th cranial nerve	**B**oth	**B**ig
10th cranial nerve	**B**oth	**B**oobs
11th cranial nerve	**M**otor	**M**atter
12th cranial nerve	**M**otor	**M**ore

* **S**= **S**ensory only/**M**=**M**otor only/**B**=**B**oth sensory & motor

24. Branchial arches: cranial nerve innervation

☑ The cranial nerves with **B**'s in the above mnemonic also give **B**ranchial arches

But (CN- 5) : 1st arch
Brother (CN-7) : 2nd arch
Big (CN-9) : 3rd arch
Boobs (CN-10) : 4th arch

25. Cranial nerve nuclei : Functional Classification [BDC-III-260]

Efferent:

1. **S**omatic **E**fferent (SE):
   <A HOT Side **E**ffect>
   A- **A**bducent nucleus
   H- **H**ypoglossal nucleus
   O- **O**cculomotor nucleus
   T- **T**rochlear nucleus
   (By **S**ide **E**ffect remember **S**omatic **E**fferent)
2. **G**eneral **V**isceral **E**fferent (GVE):
   <**G**eneral **V**isceral **E**fferent **S**aves **L**ife>
   G- (nothing)
   V- **V**agus (dorsal nucleus)
   E- **E**dinger-Westphal nucleus
   S- **S**alivary nucleus
   L- **L**acrimal nucleus
3. Special Visceral Efferent:
   <5, 7, 9-11>
   5- Motor nucleus of trigeminal nerve

7- Facial nerve nucleus
9 to 11 – Nucleus Ambiguous

Afferent:
1. Special Somatic Afferent (SSA):
Cochlear & Vestibular nuclei (VIII)
2. General Somatic Afferent (GSA):
Trigeminal nerve related nuclei (V)
- Main sensory nucleus of trigeminal nerve
- Mesencephalic nucleus of trigeminal nerve
- Spinal nucleus of trigeminal nerve

3. Visceral Afferent (VA):
Nucleus of solitary tract

☑ Remember the afferents as **<Cor-Ti-Sol>**
Cor – Cochlear & Vestibular
Ti – Trigeminal
Sol – Solitary tract

☑ Note there is no classification into general and special for **S**omatic **E**fferent & **V**isceral **A**fferent. Remember as **<No special SEVA>**

26. Nucleus Tractus Solitarius (NTS): [Gray's 38th-1018]

<**NTS**>
NTS receives afferent fibers from **N**inth, **T**enth and **S**eventh cranial nerves.

27. Cerebellar Deep Nuclei

<**L**adies **D**emand **E**xceptional **G**enerosity **F**rom **M**en>
The 4 nuclei, from lateral to medial:
[**L**ateral]
Dentate
Emboliform
Globose
Fastigial
[**M**edial]
Or simply remember : **<DEFG>**

28. Limbic System: Constituent Parts [BDC-III-275]

<**O**lfa **HAS A CUP**>

1. **O**lfactory nerves, bulb, tract, striae & trigone
2. **H**ippocampal formation (including hippocampus, the dentate gyrus, the indusium griseum & longtidunal striae)
3. **A**nterior perforated substance
4. **S**eptal region
5. **A**mygdaloid nucleus
6. **C**ingulate gyrus
7. **U**ncus
8. **P**arahippocampal gyrus

29. Venous Sinuses of Dura mater: [BDC-III-72]

Paired Venous Sinuses:

<**M**en in **T**rans **S**ing **P**arty **S**ongs **I**n **P**eter's **C**ar>

1. Middle meningeal sinus
2. Transverse sinus
3. Sigmoid sinus
4. Petrosal sinus (Superior & inferior)
5. Sphenoparietal sinus
6. Petrosquamus sinus
7. Cavernous sinus

Unpaired Venous Sinuses:

<I' BOSS">

1. Intercavernous sinus (anterior & posterior)
2. Basilar plexus of veins
3. Occipital sinus
4. Straight sinus
5. Saggital sinus (superior & inferior)

30. Cavernous sinus: Tributaries [BDC-III-73]

<**O**nly **C**entre **I**n **S**iberia **S**elling **F**resh tea>

From orbit:	**O-O**pthalmic vein
	C-Central vein
From the brain:	**I-I**nferior cerebral vein
	S-Superficial middle cerebral vein

From the meninges: **S**-**S**phenoparietal sinus
F-**F**rontal trunk of middle meningeal vein

Tea – helps you to remember that this mnemonic is for Tributaries.

31. Cavernous Sinus : Draining channels [BDC-III-73]

<**TIP F**or **I**diots>

Transverse sinus - through superior petrosal sinus
Internal jugular vein
Pterygoid plexus of veins
Facial vein – through superior ophthalmic vein
Intercavernous sinus

☑ All communications are valveless and blood can flow in either direction.

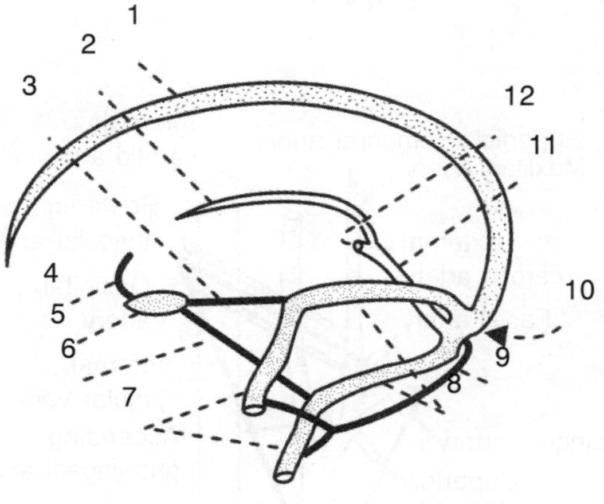

Fig 1.16: Scheme to show the intracranial venous sinuses. Lateral view (1) Superior sagittal sinus (2) Inferior sagittal sinus (3) Superior petrosal sinus (4) Sphenoparietal sinus (5) Cavernous sinus (6) Inferior petrosal sinus (7) Sigmoid sinuses (8) Transverse sinuses (9) Occipital sinus (10) Confluence of sinuses (11) Straight sinus (12) Great cerebral vein (Vein of Galen)

32. **External Carotid Artery Branches [BDC-III-103, Fig.-8.11]**

<**S**exy **L**adies **F**ollow **O**nly **P**assionate **A**nd **S**exy **M**en>

Anterior: **S**uperior thyroid
Lingual
Facial

Posterior: **O**ccipital
Posterior auricular

Medial: **A**scending pharyngeal

Terminal: **S**uperficial temporal
Maxillary

Alternatively: <**A**s **S**he **L**ay **F**lat, **O**scar's **P**assion **S**lowly **M**ounted>
<**S**ister **L**ucy's **P**owdered **F**ace **O**ften **A**ttracts **M**edical **S**tudents>
<**MAPS OF S**hri-**L**anka>
<**S**ome **A**ngry **L**ady **F**igured **O**ut **PMS**>

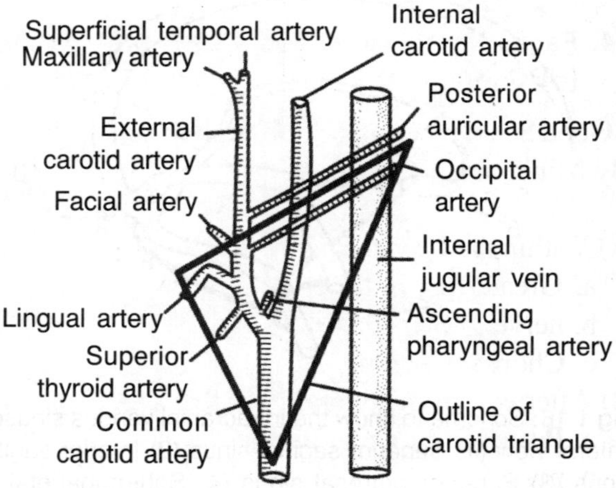

Fig 1.17: Carotid arteries, branches of the external carotid artery, and the internal jugular vein, in relation to the carotid triangle

33. Carotid sheath contents: [BDC-III-53]

<**I See 10 CC** in the **IV**>
I See (IC) = **I**nternal **C**arotid artery
10 = **10th** cranial nerve (Vagus nerve)
CC = **C**ommon **C**arotid artery
IV = **I**nternal Jugular **V**ein

☑ Ansa cervicalis nerve lies in the anterior wall of the sheath.
☑ Sympathetic chain lies posterior to the sheath.

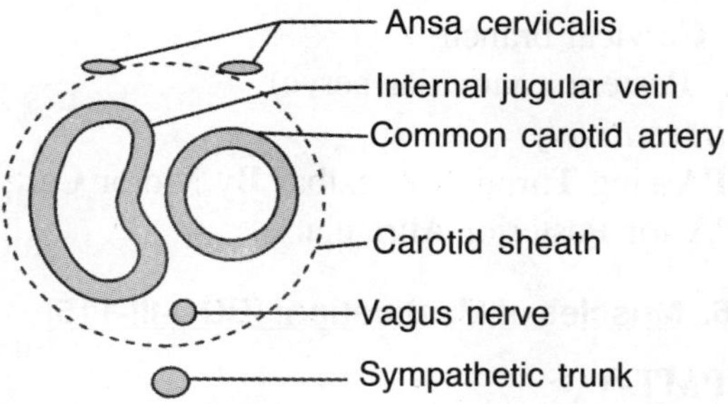

Fig 1.18: Right carotid sheath with its contents

34. Facial Nerve: Branches & Distribution [BDC-III-113]

<**G**ood **S**cholars **C**an **P**ass **D**ifficult **S**chool **T**ests **Z**ust **B**y **M**inimal **C**heating>

A) Within the Facial canal:
   a. **G**reater petrosal nerve
   b. nerve to **S**tapedius
   c. **C**horda tympani
B) After exit from stylomastoid foramen:
   a. **P**osterior auricular nerve
   b. posterior belly of **D**igastric
   c. **S**tylohyoid
C) Terminal branches:
   a. **T**emporal branch
   b. **Z**ygomatic branch

c. **B**uccal branch
d. **M**andibular branch
e. **C**ervical branch

35. Facial Nerve: Terminal Branches [BDC-III-113]

<**T**en **Z**ulus **B**uchered **M**y **C**at >
From superior to inferior:
1. **T**emporal branch
2. **Z**ygomatic branch
3. **B**uccal branch
4. **M**andibular branch
5. **C**ervical branch
6. (**P**osterior auricular nerve)

Alternatively:
<**PA**ssing **T**hrough **Z**anzibar **B**y **M**otor **C**ar>
(PA for Posterior Auricular).

36. Muscles of Mastication: [BDC-III-115]

<PMT-V_3>
Pterygoid (Lateral & medial)
Masseter
Temporalis
Supplied by **V_3** (Mandibular nerve)
☑ Develop from mesoderm of 1st branchial arch.

37. Otic ganglion: [BDC-III-127]

<All P's>
- **P**eripheral **P**arasympathetic ganglion
- supply **P**arotid gland (via. Auriculotemporal nerve)
- **P**resent medial to Mandibular nerve… but…
- **P**art of Glossopharyngeal nerve
- lesser **P**etrosal nerve forms **P**arasympathetic root
- **P**lexus on middle meningeal artery forms sympathetic root
- **P**rovides alternative pathway for taste sensation

38. Basal Ganglia: Parts [Ganong 19th-204]

<**C**unning **P**eople **G**et **S**ure **S**uccess>

'Basal Ganglia' term is generally applied to 5 structures on each side of the brain . These include:

1. Caudate nucleus
2. Putamen
3. Globus pallidus
4. Subthalamic nucleus
5. Substantia nigra

Remember:

☑ Lesion in striatum (Caudate nucleus± Putamen) leads to - *Chorea*

☑ Lesion in globus pallidus leads to - *Athetosis*

☑ Lesion in subthalamic nucleus leads to - *Hemiballismus*

☑ Lesion in substantia nigra leads to - *Parkinsonism*

39. <u>Lentiform Nucleus: Parts [BDC-III-282]</u>

<**LPG**>

Lentiform nucleus has 2 parts:

a. **P**utamen

b. **G**lobus pallidus

Also in LPG, **L** is near **P** so Putamen is Lateral

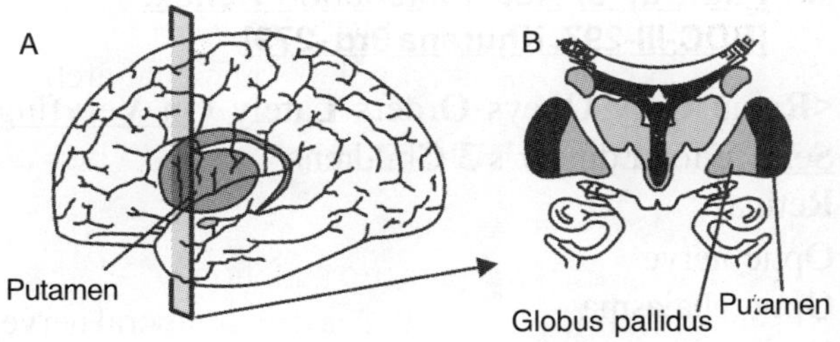

Fig. 1.19

40. <u>Commisural Fibers in the Brain: [BDC-III-284]</u>

<**H**e **H**as **F**ormed **A** **P**ublic **C**ommision>

H- Habenular commisure

H- Hypothalamic commisure

F- commisure of the **F**ornix (hippocampal commisure)
A- **A**nterior commisure
P- **P**osterior commisure
C- **C**orpus Callosum

41. Pathway of Light Reflex: [BDC-III-297, Khurana 3rd -279]

<**R**amu **O**nly **O**beys **O**rders to **L**ate **P**rince **E**dinger & **3** **C**hildren>
Retina
Optic nerve
Optic chaiasma
Optic tract
Lateral geniculate body
Pretectal nucleus
Edinger-Westphal nucleus
3rd nerve
3C's – **C**iliary ganglion
short **C**iliary nerve
Constrictor pupilae

☑ To remember that the ciliary nerve is 'short' think of children who are 'small'.

42. Pathway of Accommodation Reflex: [BDC-III-297, Khurana 3rd -279]

<**R**amu **O**nly **O**beys **O**rders **L**ately **O**n **V**eryfing **S**ervice for **E**dinger's **3** **C**hildren>
Retina
Optic nerve
Optic chaiasma
Optic tract
Lateral geniculate body
Optic radiation
Visual cortex
Superior longitudinal association tract
Edinger-Westphal nucleus
3rd nerve
3C's – **C**iliary ganglion
Ciliary muscle
Constrictor pupilae

43. Difference between Pathway of Light reflex & Accommodation reflex:

Light reflex	*Accommodation reflex*
Pretectal nucleus	**O**ptic radiation
	Visual cortex
	Superior longitudinal association tract

44. Openings in the Meatuses of Nose. [BDC-197]

<**I**diots **N**ever **M**ake **F**ast & **E**asy **M**oney, **S**aid **E**instein.>

I- **I**nferior meatus
- **N**asolacrimal duct

M- **M**iddle meatus
-**F**rontal air sinuses
-anterior **E**thmoidal air sinuses
-**M**axillary air sinuses

S- **S**uperior meatus
-posterior **E**thmiodal air sinuses

45. Little's Area (Kiesselbach's Plexus): [S. K. Dey-6th – 188]

<**A**unt **E**lisa makes **G**reat **S**upper **P**late with **S**uper **L**ove>

- **A**nterior **E**thmoidal artery
- **G**reater **P**alatine artery

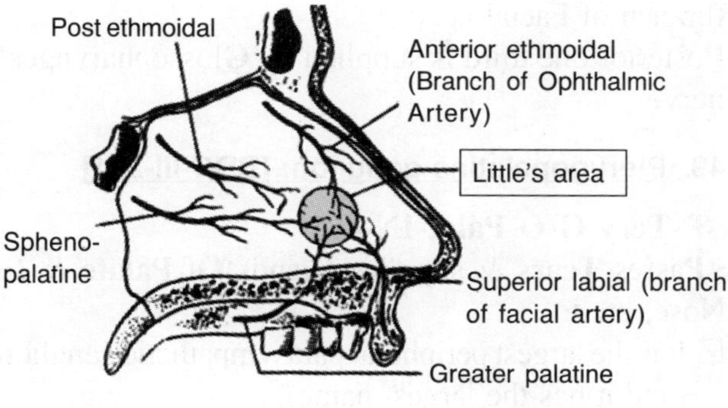

Fig. 1.20: Little's area of the nasal septum showing vascular anastomosis

- **S**pheno**P**alatine artery
- **S**uperior **L**abial artery (septal branch)

☑ It is the commonest site of epistaxis (nose bleed).

46. Safety muscle of the tongue: [Gray's 38th 1725]

<**G**entle**G**uys are safe>
Safety muscle of the tongue is **G**enio**g**lossus

47. Taste Sensation Distribution [Ganong 20th-184]

a. Bitter: Back of tongue
   -When you take a bitter pill you throw it in your mouth as far as possible.
b. Sour: On sides
   -Imagine the juice of a lemon trickling by the sides of your tongue.
c. Salty: Dorsum of tongue (anteriorly)
   -Imagine taking a pinch of salt and sprinkling it on your tongue.
d. Sweet: At the tip
   -Imagine licking a sweet candy with the tip of your tongue.

48. Taste Pathway: [Ganong 20th-184]

<**A**nyone **C**an **P**ass **G**as !>
Anterior two third is supplied by **C**horda Tympani (branch of Facial nerve)
Posterior one third is supplied by **G**lossopharyngeal nerve

49. Pterygopalatine ganglion: [BDC-III-201]

<P-Tery-G-O-Palat-IN-e >
<**P**asses **Tears** & supplies **G**lands **O**f **Palate** & **In** **N**ose, etc.>

☑ It is the largest peripheral parasympathetic ganglion (and it has the largest name).

☑ It supplies secretomotor fibers to the lacrimal gland, palate, mucous glands of nose & paranasal sinuses, pharynx.
☑ It is also called sphenopalatine ganglion as it lies close to the sphenopalatine foramen in the pterygopalatine fossa.
☑ **M**aximum **F**orgotten point about the ganglion: It is related to the **M**axillary nerve but it is functionally connected to the **F**acial nerve (through greater petrosal branch).

50. Foramen Spinosum Transmits : [BDC-III-24]

<Spinning Meningeal VAN>
- Middle meningeal **v**ein (posterior trunk)
- Middle meningeal **a**rtery
- Meningeal branch of mandibular **n**erve (nervous spinosus)

51. Spinal Cord: Facts

Spinal Cord is made up of **31** segments.
In children it ends upto **L3** & in adults it ends in **L1.**

☑ *Also remember:*
Spinal cord segments are :
8 cervical
12 thoracic
5 lumbar
5 sacral
1 coccyxigeal

52. Subarachnoid Space: Level

< **S**ubarachnoid **S**pace **(S+S = S2)** >
The subarachnoid space extends to the lower border of S2.

53. Bones in the Orbit of Eye: [BDC-III-22]

This mnemonic relies on the belief that a species called the **FLEZMS** are in **ORBIT** around the earth.
F: Frontal
L: Lacrimal

E: **E**thmoid
Z: **Z**ygomatic
M: **M**axilla
S: **S**phenoid

54. Extraocular Muscles Cranial Nerve Innervation

<LR6 SO4 rest **3>**
Lateral Rectus is supplied by 6th nv.
Superior Oblique is supplied by 4th nv.
Rest are all supplied by 3rd cranial nerve.

55. Extra ocular muscles [BDC-III-86]

<SIN RAD>
Superiors are **In**torters
Rectus are **Ad**ductors

56. Cranial Bones

<PEST OF 6>
1. Parietal
2. Ethmoid
3. Sphenoid
4. Temporal
5. Occipital
6. Frontal
6 = number of bones

Alternatively:
"**O**ld **P**eople **F**rom **T**exas **E**at **S**piders"
☑ The skull contains total 22 bones.

57. Lymphoid organs: Primary and Secondary [Gray's 38th-1423]

Primary:
There are 2 types of lymphocytes **T and B.**
So there are 2 primary lymphoid organs **Thymus and Bone marrow**.

Secondary:
Lymph nodes

Spleen
Tonsils
Appendix.
Mucosa-associated lymphoid tissue or MALT

58. Cartilages of the Larynx

There are 4 cartilages in the larynx are
<CEAT>

- **C**ricoid
- **E**piglottis
- **A**rytenoid
- **T**hyroid

59. Naso-lacrimal Duct: [BDC-III-49]

<**Hasner** has **Inferiority** complex because he became **BALD** at **18**>

- Nasolacrimal duct is directed **Ba**ckwards, **L**aterally and **D**ownwards.
- A fold of mucous membrane forms an imperfect valve at the lower end – Valve of **Hasner**
- It **18 mm** long.
- Opens in the **inferior** meatus.

60. Styloid Apparatus: [BDC-III-166]

The styloid process with the structures attached to it is called the styloid apparatus.
The five attachments resemble the **Reins of a Chariot.**

1. Stylohyoid muscle – 2nd arch derivative (Facial nerve supply)
2. Stylohyoid ligament- 2nd arch derivative
3. Stylo**pharyngeus** muscle – 3rd arch derivative (glosso**pharyngeal** nerve supply)
4. Stylo**glossus** – Supplied by hypo**glossal** nerve.
5. Stylo**M**andibular ligament –Remnant of dorsal part of **M**eckel's cartilage.

I. MISCELLANEOUS

61. Deep Tendon Reflexes: Root Supply

God designed body reflexes according to a nursery rhyme:

<One, two— buckle my shoe.
Three, four— kick the door.
Five, six— pick up sticks.
Seven, eight— shut the gate >

S1,2 = ankle jerk
L3,4 = knee jerk
C5,6 = biceps and brachioradialis
C7,8 = triceps jerk

62. Joints in the Midline

<SC>

In medial line, below Second Cervical, joints are Secondary Cartilaginous and usually have a diSC.

☑ Note: Secondary cartilaginous is also known as symphysis.

☑ The one that doesn't have a disc is xiphi-sternal

63. Ossification Ages [Reddy-59]

<**E**very **P**otential **A**natomist **S**hould **K**now **W**hen>

When they ossify, in order of increasing year:

Elbow: 16 years
Pelvis, **A**nkle: 17 years
Shoulder, **K**nee: 18 years
Wrist: 19 years

64. Vertebrae: Recognizing A Thoracic from Lumbar

Examine vertebral body shape:

Thoracic vertebra has heart-shaped body since your heart is in your thorax.

Lumbar vertebra has kidney-bean shaped since kidneys are in lumbar area.

65. Teratogenesis: When It Occurs [IBS-361]

TEratogenesis is most likely during organogenesis—between the:

Third and **E**ighth weeks of gestation (embryonic period)

66. Weeks 2, 3, 4 of Development: An Event for each [IBS-41]

Week **Two**: **Bi**laminar germ disc.
Week **Three**: **Tri**laminar germ disc.
Week **Four**: **Four** limbs appear.

67. Pharyangeal Arches: Nerve Supply [IBS-115]

<**M**andi's **F**ather **G**oes **S**hopping **R**egularly>

1st Arch — **M**andibular nerve
2nd Arch — **F**acial nerve
3rd Arch — **G**lossopharyngeal nerve
4th Arch — **S**uperior Laryngeal nerve
5th arch — *disappears.*
6th Arch — **R**ecurrant Laryngeal Nerve

68. Cartilage Derivatives of 1st Pharyngeal Arch (Mandibular)

<**I'M A S**uper **S**exy **G**uy>

1. **I**ncus
2. **M**alleus
3. **A**nterior ligament of malleus
4. **S**pine of sphenoid
5. **S**phenomandibular ligament
6. **G**enial tubercle of mandible

69. Structures Derived from Neural Crest: [I.B. Singh-5th – 321]

<**N**o **CAMPS D**ear !>

1. **N**eurons*
2. **C**hromaffin cells in adrenal medulla
3. **A**rachnoid mater
4. **M**elanoblasts
5. **P**ia mater

6. **S**chwan cells
7. **D**ental papilla (Odontoblasts differentiate from the cells of the dental papilla)

☑ The neurons are:
- spinal posterior nerve root ganglia (dorsal root ganglia)
- sensory ganglia of the 5th ,7th ,8th ,9th ,10th cranial nerves
- sympathetic ganglia

☑ The neural crest are bilaterally paired strips of cells arising in the ectoderm at the margins of the neural tube. These cells migrate to many different locations and differentiate into many cell types within the embryo.

☑ Failure of neural crest cells to migrate will result in anomalies such as albinism, elephant man, or oropharyngeal teratoma etc.

70. Gastrulation: [Langman's Medical Embryology 8th-61]

- All **3** germ layers are established in…
- **3**rd week of embryo
  This prosess is called gastrulation.

71. Bifurcation Vertebral Landmarks

A bifurcation occurs on 4th level of each vertebral column:

C4: bifurcation of Common carotid artery
T4: bifurcation of Trachea
L4: bifurcation of Aorta

72. Hyaline vs. Elastic Cartilage [Gray's Anatomy 38th – 452]

Yellow elastic cartilage:

<Cry **AEEEE**… when your ear is pulled.>

1. **C**orniculate cartilage
2. **A**pices of the arytenoids
3. **E**xternal ear
4. **E**ustaschian tube
5. **E**piglottis

6. **E**xternal auditory canal

Hy**al**ine cartilage:
All cartilage names ending in '**al**'.
1. Cost**al**
2. Nas**al**
3. Laryngе**al**
4. Tracheobronchi**al**
5. **Al**l temporary and most articular cartilages

73. Structures Containing No Lymphatics: [gray's 35th-714]

<BABES>
Brain and spinal cord
Avascular structures (Hair, nail cornea, articular cartilages)
Bone marrow
Epidermis
Splenic pulp

74. Centromere arrangement in chromosomes:

<M-SAT>
Metacentric
Submetacentric
Acrocentric
Telocentric
Alternatively: <MAST>

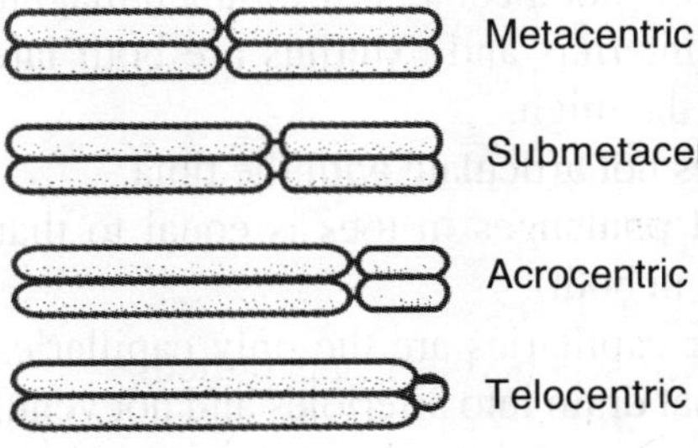

Fig. 1.21

75. Centromere Location in X and Y chromosome: [Molecular genetics by Precid and Strachan /49, 153]

Mnemonic *in hindi:* <**X** hi **Sub** hai ? …**YA**! >
Human **X** chromosome is large **Sub**metacentric chromosome with numerous genes.
Human **Y** chromosome is a small **A**crocentric chromosome.

76. True Ribs: [BDC-I-157]

There are seven true ribs (1 to 7)
Se**V**en ribs attach to both **S**ternum and **V**ertebra.

77. Length of Organs:

<FUDO is 25>
Length of **F**ilum terminale, **U**reter, **D**uodenum & **O**esophagus is **25** cm

78. Liver Segments : [Sabiston 16th-1000]

Li**V**er is divided into segments by **2 V**eins – **Hepatic Vein** and **Portal Vein**. (Fig. 122).

79. Planter Vs. Dorsi Flexion

PLANTar flexion of foot – is what you do when you squash a **PLANT** with your foot.

80. Know These Wonders in Anatomy

1. Spinal cord is not a content of foramen magnum.
2. Obturator internus and externus are both lateral rotators of the thigh.
3. Patella does not articulate with the tibia.
4. Number of phalanges in toes is equal to that in fingers (14 in both).
5. Glomerular capillaries are the only capillaries in the body that drain into arterioles and not venules.
6. Facial nerve passes through but does not give any branch to parotid.
7. Optic nerve is not a content of supra orbital fissure.

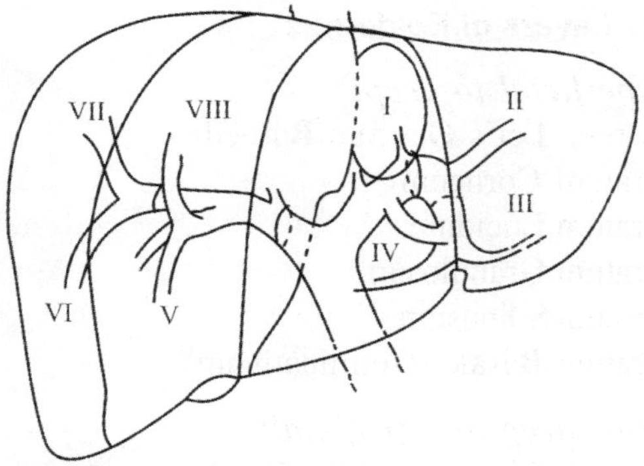

The French System

(couinoud and colleagues)

- The system shows more considerations for the hepatic venous drainage and caudate lobe but also applies to the portal anatomy.
- The planes containing the right, middle and left *hepatic veins* are called portal scissurae whereas planes containing the *portal pedicles* are called the hepatic scissurae.
- They divide liver into eight segments.

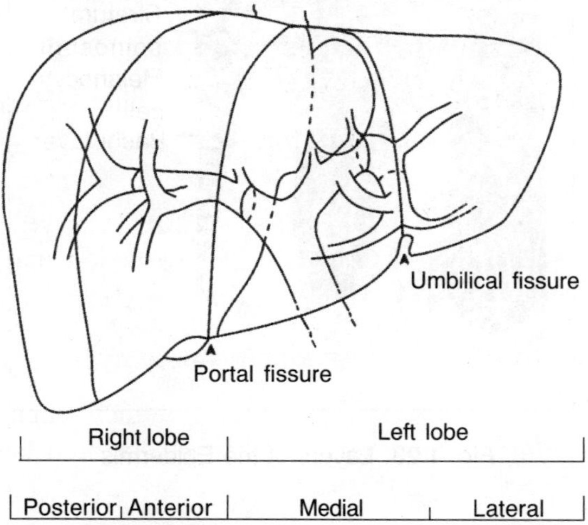

The American System

- The general relationship between hepatic veins and portal vein branches is used to determine the lobar anatomy of the liver.
- They divided liver into four segments.

Fig. 1.22: Anatomy of hepatic lobes can be elaborated two systems of segmental nomenclature

81. Layers of Epidermis

Superficial to deep:
<**C**ome **L**et’s **G**et **S**un **B**urned>
Stratum **C**orneum
Stratum **L**ucidum
Stratum **G**ranulosum
Stratum **S**pinosum
Stratum **B**asale (**G**erminativum)

From deep to superficial:
<**G**ood **S**kin **G**lows **L**ike **C**andle>

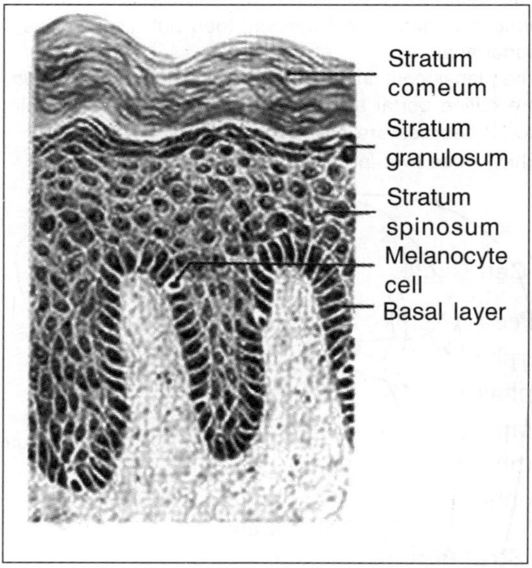

Fig. 1.23: Layers of the Epidermis

82. Some Commonly Asked Relationships:

i. At the hilum of kidney – *(from ant. to post.)*
- Renal **v**ein
- Renal **a**rtery [VAP]
- Renal **p**elvis

ii. At the femoral triangle – *(from medial to lateral)*
- Femoral **v**ein
- Femoral **a**rtery [VAN]
- Femora] **n**erve

iii. At the intercostal groove — *(from above downwards)*
- Intercostal **v**ein
- Intercostal **a**rtery [VAN]
- Intercostal **n**erve

iv. At the popliteal fossa:
- In upper part – *(from medial to lateral)*
  - Popliteal **a**rtery
  - Popliteal **v**ein
  - Tibial **n**erve [AVN]
- In middle part – *(from superficial to deep)*
  - Tibial **n**erve
  - Poplitial **v**ein [NVA]
  - Popliteal **a**rtery
- In lower part – *(from medial to lateral)*
  - Tibial **n**erve
  - Popliteal **v**ein [NVA]
  - Popliteal **a**rtery

v. In cubital fossa – *(from medial to lateral)*
- **M**edian nerve
- **B**rachial artery (MBBR)
- **B**iceps tendon
- **R**adial nerve.

83. Cell Cycle:

<**I P**ee (on the) **M.A.T.**>
Interphase
Prophase
Metaphase
Anaphase
Telophase

84. Stratified Squamous Cells

To remember that Stratified Squamous cells are found in two locations:
Lining the Mouth
Lining the Vagina.

One is Stratified Squamous — the other SATISFIED Squamous

85. Adult Equivalents of Embryonic Structures

See next page

Embryonic structure	*Male*	*Female*
Indifferent gonad	Testis	Ovary
Cortex	Seminiferous tubules	Ovarian follicles
Medulla	Rete testis	Rete ovarii
Gubernaculum	Gubernaculum testis	Ovarian and round ligament of uterus
Mesonephric tubules	Ductuli efferentes	Epoophoron Paroophoron
Mesonephric duct	Appendix of epididymus Duct of epididymus Ductus deferens Ureter Calices and collecting tubules Ejaculatory duct Seminal vesicles	Appendix vesiculosa Duct of epoophoron Duct of gartner Ureter Pelvis Calices Collecting tubules
Paramesonephric duct	Appendix of testis	Hydatid of morgagni Uterine tube Uterus
Urogenital sinus	Urinary bladder Urethra Prostatic utricle Prostate gland Bulbourethral glands	Urinary bladder Urethra Vagina Urethral Paraurethral Greater vestibular glands
Sinus tubercle	Seminal colliculus	Hymen
Phallus	Penis	Clitoris
Urogenital folds	Ventral aspect of penis	Labia minora
Labioscrotal swellings	Scrotum	Labia majora

86. Quick Peritoneum Facts

The idea is to relate key letters of related parts. E.g., stomach and omentum (which lays over the stomach) share the letters OM.

- The **Omentum** covers the stomach
- The **Lesser Omentum** holds the Liver and stomach

- The **Mesentery** holds the s<u>m</u>all intestine
- The **mesoCOLON** attaches the large intestine (colon) to the posterior abdominal wall
- The **PERITONEUM,** holds PERson's Intestines To Nearest wall.
- The bacterium **E. coli** is found in Everybody's Colon

87. PPL's Tonsils

People (PPL for short) have 3 tonsils: **Pharyngeal, Palatine, and Lingual**.

MULTIPLE CHOICE QUESTIONS

1. **Vaginal epithelium is derived from:**
   A. Mesoderm of genital ridge
   B. Endoderm of genital ridge
   C. Mesoderm of urogenital sinus
   D. Endoderm of urogenital sinus
2. **Which of the following is not the part of ethmoid bone?**
   A. Agger nasi
   B. Crista galli
   C. Uncinate process
   D. Inferior turbinate
3. **Which part of the fallopian tube acts as a functional/ anatomical sphincter?**
   A. Isthmus
   B. Intramural
   C. Ampulla
   D. Infundibulum
4. **Most important blood supply to stomach:**
   A. Left gastric artery
   B. Short gastric artery
   C. Right gastro epiploic artery
   D. Left gastro epiploic artery
5. **"Dynamic stabilizer of shoulder joint" term is used for:**
   A. Rotator cuff
   B. Glenoid labrum
   C. Coracohumeral ligament
   D. Glenohumeral ligament
6. **Which of the following is not a derivative of neural ectoderm?**
   A. Sphincter pupillae
   B. Retina
   C. Dilator pupillae
   D. Ciliary muscles

7. **Muscle, which is anatomically a back muscle, but functionally related to thorax is:**
   A. Rhomboid
   B. Latisimus dorsi
   C. Trapezius
   D. Levator costae
8. **Which of the following artery does not supply medulla?**
   A. Anterior spinal artery
   B. Vertebral artery
   C. Posterior inferior cerebellar artery
   D. Superior cerebellar artery
9. **External anal sphincter is innervated by:**
   A. S2, S3, S4
   B. S2, S3
   C. L5, S1
   D. L2, L3
10. **Nerve root for dermatome supplying thumb and index finger:**
    A. C6 C7
    B. C6 C6
    C. C7 C8
    D. C5 C6
11. **A patient woke up with difficulty in extending fingers, can make a grip and hold a pen. Dorsiflexon was normal. Sensory and motor examination was normal. Nerve most commonly involved:**
    A. C8T1
    B. Posterior interosseous nerve
    C. Lower brachial plexus
    D. Hand area in cortex
12. **Regular vein, artery and nerve ("VAN") arrangement is not present in which intercostal space (not the rib):**
    A. First intercostal space
    B. Second intercostal space

C. Third intercostal space
D. Eleventh intercostal space

13. **Which of the following is not enclosed in mesorectal fascia?**
A. Pararectal nodes
B. Superior rectal vein
C. Inferior rectal vein
D. Inferior mesenteric plexus

14. **In spermatogenesis, independent assortment of paternal and maternal chromosomes occurs during:**
A. Primary to secondary spermatocyte
B. Spermatogonia to primary spermatocyte
C. Secondary spermatocyte to spermatids
D. Spermatids to spermatozoa

15. **Major and most powerful muscle of the rotator cuff which has an enormous meaning in the gleno-humeral stability and it is neglected in the clinical literature. Forgotten muscle in rotator cuff shoulder, which was not given importance earlier in regard to dislocation of shoulder but now coming back in focus:**
A. Supraspinatus
B. Infraspinatus
C. Teres minor
D. Subscapularis

16. **Which of the following structure is not present at floor of third ventricle?**
A. Optic stalk
B. Third nerve
C. Infundibulum
D. Mamillary body

17. **Boundaries of facial recess are formed by all of the following except:**
A. Facial nerve
B. Stapedius tendon
C. Chorda tympani
D. Short process of incus

18. Elevation at the urethral crest in prostatic urethra is elevation formed by:
A. Prostatic glands
B. Elongation of detrusor
C. Trigone muscle attachment
D. Preprostatic internal sphincter

19. Which of the following is not a component of anorectal ring?
A. External anal sphincter
B. Puborectalis
C. Anococcygeal raphe
D. Internal anal sphincter

20. Inferior wall of orbit is formed by all of the following except:
A. Ethmoid
B. Maxillary
C. Palatine
D. Zygomatic

21. Lacrimation is lost due to lesion of:
A. Nasociliary nerve
B. Greater petrosal nerve
C. Trigeminal nerve
D. Anterior ethmoidal nerve

22. All of the following structures are pierced in pleural fluid aspiration except:
A. Skin
B. Thoracic fascia
C. Pulmonary pleura
D. Intercostal muscles

23. Complete cartilage ring is seen in:
A. Cricoid cartilage
B. Thyroid cartilage
C. Cunieform cartilage
D. Epiglottis

24. Vaginal epithelium is derived from:
A. Mesoderm of genital ridge
B. Endoderm of genital ridge
C. Mesoderm of urogenital sinus
D. Endoderm of urogenital sinus

25. The architecture of the liver is divided into lobes by:
A. Bile duct
B. Hepatic artery
C. Hepatic vein
D. Portal vein
E. Lymphatics

26. Branches of anterior division of internal iliac artery:
A. Superior gluteal artery
B. Obturatory artery
C. Uterine artery
D. Iliolumbar artery
E. Internal pudenal artery

27. Lacrimal gland is supplied by which of the following ganglia?
A. Otic ganglia
B. Ciliary ganglion
C. Spenopalatine ganglion
D. Submandibular ganglion

28. Following structures passing through CARPAL TUNNEL *except:*
A. FDP
B. FD superficialis
C. FP longus
D. Palmaris longus

29. True about gastrulation is:
A. Process involving rotation of gastrointestinal tract
B. Process by which three germinal layers form
C. Occurs in 4th week of gestation
D. Involves hypoblastic inner cell mass

30. Oligodendrocytes are important in:
A. Blood brain barrier
B. Myelin formation
C. Phagocytosis
D. Chemotaxis

31. Which is not the content of the femoral sheath?

A. Femoral nerve
B. Femoral artery
C. Femoral vein
D. Deep inguinal node

32. A person has inability to look downward and laterally. The nerve injured is:
A. Occulomotor
B. Trochlear
C. Abducent
D. Trigeminal

33. A posteriorly perforating ulcer in the pyloric antrum of the stomach is most likely to produce initial localized peritonitis or abscess formation in the following:
A. Omental bursa (lesser sac)
B. Greater sac
C. Right subphrenic space
D. Hepato renal space (pouch of Morison)

34. Injury to radial in lower part of spiral groove:
A. Spares nerve supply to extensor carpi radialis longus
B. Results in paralysis of anconeus muscle
C. Leaves extensions at elbow joint intact
D. Weakness pronation movement

35. The most common variation in the arteries arising from the arch of aorta is:
A. Absence of brachiocephalic trunk
B. Left vertebral artery arising from the arch
C. Left common carotid artery arising from brachiocephalic trunk
D. Presence of retroesophageal subclavian artery

36. After radical mastectomy there was injury to the long thoracic nerve. The integrity of the nerve can be tested at the bedside by asking the patient to:
A. Shrug the shoulders
B. Raise the arm above the head on the affected side

C. Touch the opposite shoulder
D. Lift a heavy object from the ground

37. **Infection/inflammation of all of the following, causes enlarged superficial inguinal lymph nodes *except*:**
A. Isthmus of uterine tube
B. Inferior part of anal canal
C. Big toe
D. Penile urethra

38. **Recurrent laryngeal nerve is in close association with:**
A. Superior thyroid artery
B. Inferior thyroid artery
C. Middle thyroid artery
D. Superior thyroid artery

39. **A 40-year-old tailor complains of pain, numbness and weakness of the right hand for the last three months. On examination, there is hypoasthesia and atrophy of thenar eminence. Which one of the following nerves is likely to be involved?**
A. Ulnar
B. Radial
C. Axillary
D. Median

40. **The type of joint between the sacrum and the coccyx is a:**
A. Symphysis
B. Syostosis
C. Synchondrosis
D. Syndesmosis

41. **Which of the following nuclei belongs to the general visceral efferent column?**

A. Facial nerve nucleus
B. Trigeminal motor nucleus
C. Dorsal nucleus of vagus
D. Nucleus ambiguous

42. **Trendelenburg's sign is positive with weakness/paralysis:**
A. Gluteus maximus

B. Gluteus medius and minimus
C. Adductor longus
D. Hamstrings

43. The anterior cruciate ligament of knee joint:
A. Prevents backward displacement of tibial condyles
B. Prevents forward displacement of tibial condyles
C. Is attached above to the medial femoral condyle
D. Prevents side to side displacement of the tibial condyles

44. Major function of gluteus medius and minimus at hip joint is:
A. Flexion
B. Extension
C. Abduction
D. Adduction

45. Opening of jaw is done by:
A. Masseter
B. Temporalis
C. Medial pterygoid
D. Lateral pterygoid

46. The following are the contents of spermatic cord *except*:
A. Genital branch of genito femoral
B. Ilioinguinal nerve
C. Testicular artery
D. Cremasteric artery

47. Lymphatics are found in:
A. Brain
B. Internal ear
C. Dermis
D. Choroid

48. Nasolacrimal duct is directed:
A. Downward, medially, backwards
B. Downwards, laterally, backwards
C. Downwards, laterally, forward
D. Downward, medially, forward

49. The most common variation in the arteries arising from the arch of aorta is:
A. Absence of brachiocephalic trunk
B. Left vertebral artery arising from the arch
C. Left common carotid artery arising from brachiocephalic trunk
D. Presence of retroesophageal subclavian artery

50. Basal ganglion contains all *except*:
A. Globus pallidus
B. Putamen
C. Thalamus
D. Letinoform nucleus

51. Median nerve supplies:
A. Abductor pollicis longus
B. Abductor pollicis brevis
C. Adductor pollicis
D. First dorsal interossecus

52. Glans penis drains into:
A. Ext. iliac Lymph nodes
B. Deep inguinal Lymph nodes
C. Paraaortic Lymph nodes
D. Superior inguinal Lymph nodes

53. Which is direct content of cavernous sinus?
A. Ophthalmic division of trigeminal nerve
B. Trochlear nerve
C. Abducent nerve
D. Occulomotor nerve

54. Safety muscle of the tongue is:
A. Hyoglossus
B. Genoiglossus
C. Palatoglossus
D. Styloglossus

55. The secretomotor fiber to the parotid gland passes through:
A. Otic ganglion
B. Sphenopalatine ganglion
C. Geniculate ganglion
D. Lesser ganglion

56. *True* ribs are:
A. 7th rib
B. 8th rib

C. 10th rib
D. 12th rib

57. Structure passing deep to flexor retinaculam, behind medial malleolus is:
A. Tibialis anterior
B. Tibialis posterior
C. Posterior tibial artery
D. Tendon of extensor hallucis longus

58. Anterior cruciate ligament is attached to:
A. Medial part of anterior intercondylar area
B. Lateral part of medial condyle
C. Lateral part of lateral *condyle*
D. Medial surface of lateral condyle

59. Depressor's of mandible:
A. Medial pterygoid
B. Masseter
C. Lateral pterygoid
D. Temporalis

60. Manubriosternal joint:
A. Saddle type
B. Ball and socket
C. Symphysis
D. Syndesmosis

61. While flexing knee, femoral condyles are prevented from rolling backwards by:
A. Ligamentum patellae
B. Semilunar cartilages
C. Medial and lateral collateral ligaments
D. Cruciate ligaments

62. Cremasteric reflex is governed by:
A. S_1
B. L_1
C. L_4
D. S_3

63. All of the following structures are related to cavernous sinus *except*:
A. Optic nerve
B. IVth cranial nerve
C. VIth nerve
D. Maxillary division of trigeminal nerve

64. Nerve supply of brachialis is from:
A. Median nerve
B. Musculocutaneous nerve
C. Ulnar nerve
D. Posterior interosseus artery

65. Serratus anterior is supplied by:
A. Thoracodorsal nerve
B. Nerve to subclavius
C. Long thoracic nerve
D. Axillary nerve

66. Bochdalek hernia of diaphragm is through:
A. Central tendon
B. Esophagal hiatus
C. Posterolateral space
D. Retrosternal space

67. Inguinal canal is not bounded posteriorly by:
A. Transversalis fascia
B. Internal oblique
C. Conjoint tendon
D. Lacunar ligament

68. Muscle supplied by glossopharyngeal nerve is:
A. Stylopharyngeus
B. Stylohyoid
C. Styloglossus
D. Thyrohyoid

69. Structure passing through foramen spinosum:
A. Accessory meningeal artery
B. Middle meningeal artery
C. Mandibular nerve
D. Maxillary nerve

70. Which of the following umbilical vessels disappears first?
A. Left umbilical vein
B. Right umbilical vein
C. Left umblical artery
D. Right umbilical artery

71. Fibres of acoustic radiation arise in the:
A. Lateral geniculate body
B. Medial geniculate body
C. Thalamus
D. Temporal lobe

72. The action of lumbricals is:
A. Abduction at MP joint
B. Extension at MP joint
C. Flexion at MP and extension at IP joint
D. Extension at MP joint and flexion at IP joint

73. Motor nerve supply to destrusors of the bladder is:
A. L_2 L_3 L_4
B. S_1 S_2
C. S_2 S_3 S_4
D. S_4 S_5

74. Seventh, Ninth and Tenth cranial nerves end in:
A. Nucleus tractus solitarius
B. Nucleus ambiguus
C. Dorsal nucleus of vagus
D. Long tract of V nerve

75. Which is not a branch of posterior cord of Brachial plexus?
A. Lower subscapular
B. Axillary
C. Dorsal scapular
D. Thoracodorsal

76. Which is not a tributary of left renal vein?
A. Inferior phrenic
B. Left gonadal
C. First lumbar
D. Left supra renal

77. The following is not a content of broad ligament:
A. Round ligament
B. Ovarian ligament
C. Fallopian tube
D. Ovary

78. The following is true for ureter:
A. Crossed anteriorly by gonadal artery
B. Length of 50 cm
C. Nerve supply from T8 - T10
D. Crossed posteriorly by renal artery

79. Foramen magnum transmits all *except*:
A. Vertebral artery

B. Spinal branch of 11th nerve
C. Spinal cord
D. Vertebral venous plexus

80. Sphenopalatine ganglion does not supply:
A. Nasal mucosa
B. Sublingual gland
C. Ciliary ganglion
D. Palate

81. Internal organs in the fetus develop at:
A. 24 weeks
B. 12 weeks
C. 8 weeks
D. 6 weeks

82. Perineal body is formed by all *except*:
A. Levator ani muscle
B. External anal sphincter muscle
C. Bulbospongiosus muscle
D. Obturator internus muscle

83. The bed of the stomach is not formed by:
A. Left kidney
B. Left supra renal gland
C. Splenic artery
D. Tail of pancreas

84. Myelin sheath in CNS is synthesized by:
A. Microglia
B. Schwann cell
C. Oligodendroglia
D. All

85. Fibres passing through posterior column is/are:
A. Post spinocerebellar tract
B. Anterior spinocerebellar tract
C. Lateral spinothalamic tract
D. Fasciculus gracilis

86. The actions of superior oblique muscle is:
A. Abduction
B. Intorsion
C. Extrosion
D. Depression

87. Flexors of the elbow are:
A. Branchialis

B. Biceps
C. Branchioradialis
D. Coracobrachialis

88. All are nuclei of the basal ganglia *except*:
A. Caudate nucleus
B. Amydaloid nucleus
C. Lentinoform nucleus
D. Dentate nuclei

89. Housemaids knee is an inflammation of the bursa:
A. Suprapatellar
B. Semi membraneus
C. Prepatellar
D. Lateral patella

90. Labourers nerve is:
A. Median
B. Ulnar
C. Radial
D. Sciatic

91. Root value of radial nerve is:
A. $C_{5,6}$
B. $C_{4,5}$
C. $C_{5,6,7}$
D. $C_{6,7}$

92. In the new born, the spinal cord ends at:
A. L3
B. S4
C. L5
D. Ll

93. Erb's point is:
A. C_5-C_6
B. C_6-C_7
C. C_7-C_8
D. C_8-T_1

94. The structures in the free border of the lesser omentum anterior to posterior are:
A. CBD, Hepatic artery, Portal vein
B. Portal vein, Hepatic artery, CBD
C. Hepatic artery, portal vein, CBD
D. Portal vein, CBD, hepatic artery

95. Structures passing through the lesser sciatic foramen are all *except*:
A. Obturator internus tendon
B. Pudenal nerve
C. Internal pudenal vessels
D. Superior gluteal nerve

96. Which structures does not pass through the carpal tunnel?
A. Median nerve
B. Radial bursa
C. Ulnar bursa
D. Ulnar nerve

97. The spinal nerves pairs are:
A. 28
B. 30
C. 31
D. 33
E. 35

98. Parasympathetic supply to rectum and anal canal:
A. L_4 L_5 S_1
B. L_5 S_1 S_2
C. S_1 S_2 S_3
D. S_2 S_3 S_4

99. Root value of phrenic nerve:
A. C_2 C_3 C_4
B. C_1 C_2 C_3
C. C_3 C_4 C_5
D. C_4 C_5 C_6
E. C_5 C_6 C_7

100. The first bone to ossify in membrane is:
A. Scaphoid
B. Scapula
C. Clavicle
D. Fibula
E. Femur

101. The cavernous sinus communicates directly with all, *except*:
A. Inferior petrosal sinus
B. Pterygoid venous plexus
C. Veins in orbit
D. Sigmoid sinus and straight sinus

102. Skull consists of bones:
A. 20
B. 22
C. 24
D. 28

103. The left subclavian artery is a branch of:
A. Brachiocephalic trunk
B. Ascending aorta
C. Arch of aorta
D. Left common carotid

104. The only pharyngeal muscle innervated by the glossopharyngeal nerve is the:
A. Stylo pharyngeus
B. Palato pharyngeus
C. Superior constrictor
D. Middle constrictor

105. Which of the following structures is not present within the lesser omentum?
A. Portal vein
B. Bile duct
C. Inferior vena cava
D. Hepatic artery
E. Lymph nodes

106. The coracobrachialis assists in which movement of the arm:
A. Flexion
B. Extension
C. Rotation
D. Supination

107. Floor of the femoral triangle is formed by the following muscles, *except* the:
A. Pectineus
B. Adductor longus
C. Iliacus
D. Adductor brevis

108. Isthmus of the thyroid gland is across tracheal rings:
A. 2nd to 4th
B. 3rd to 5th
C. 5th and 6th
D. 4th only

109. Radial nerve 2 inches distal to the elbow joint gives:
A. Muscular branches
B. Sensory branches
C. Articular branches
D. All of the above

110. Boxer's muscle is:
A. Trapezius
B. Serratus anterior
C. Psoas major
D. Latissimus dorsi

111. Due to bony support, the most stable position of the ankle joint is:
A. Inversion
B. Plantar flexion
C. Eversion
D. Dorsiflexion

112. In walking, the hip bone of the suspended leg is raised by which of the following muscles acting on the supported side of the body?
A. Obturator externus
B. Gluteus medius
C. Gluteus maximus
D. Gluteus minimus

113. Which of the following bones does not form the proximal row of carpal *bones?*
A. Scaphoid
B. Lunate
C. Triquetral
D. Capitate

114. Nucleus in brain common to IX, X and XI cranial nerves:
A. Nucleus solitarius
B. Nucleus ambiguous
C. Dentate nucleus
D. Red nucleus

ANSWERS

1. **D.** Endoderm of urogenital sinus
2. **D.** Inferior turbinate
3. **A.** Isthmus
4. **A.** Left gastric artery
5. **A.** Rotator cuff
6. **D.** Ciliary muscles
7. **B.** Latisimus dorsi
8. **D.** Superior cerebellar artery
9. **A.** S2, S3, S4
10. **B.** C6 C6
11. **B.** Posterior interosseous nerve
12. **A.** First intercostal space
13. **C.** Inferior rectal vein
14. **A.** Primary to secondary spermatocyte
15. **D.** Subscapularis
16. **B.** Third nerve
17. **B.** Stapedius tendon
18. **A.** Prostatic glands
19. **C.** Anococcygeal raphe
20. **A.** Ethmoid
21. **B.** Greater petrosal nerve
22. **B.** Thoracic fascia
23. **A.** Cricoid cartilage
24. **D.** Endoderm of urogenital sinus
25. **C.** Hepatic vein
    D. Portal vein
26. **A.** Superior gluteal artery
    C. Uterine artery
    E. Internal pudenal artery
27. **C.** Spenopalatine ganglion
28. **D.** Palmaris longus
29. **B.** Process by which three germinal layers form
30. **B.** Myelin formation
31. **A.** Femoral nerve
32. **B.** Trochlear
33. **A.** Omental bursa (lesser sac)
34. **C.** Leaves extensions at elbow joint intact
35. **C.** Left common carotid artery arising from brachiocephalic trunk
36. **B.** Raise the arm above the head on the affected side

37. **D.** Penile urethra
38. **B.** Inferior thyroid artery
39. **D.** Median
40. **A.** Symphysis
41. **C.** Dorsal nucleus of vagus
42. **B.** Gluteus medius and minimus
43. **B.** Prevents forward displacement of tibial condyles
44. **C.** Abduction
45. **D.** Lateral pterygoid
46. **B.** Ilioinguinal nerve
47. **C.** Dermis
48. **B.** Downwards, laterally, backwards
49. **C.** Left common carotid artery arising from brachiocephalic trunk
50. **C.** Thalamus
51. **B.** Abductor pollicis brevis
52. **B.** Deep inguinal lymph nodes
53. **C.** Abducent nerve
54. **B.** Genoiglossus
55. **A.** Otic ganglion
56. **A.** 7th rib
57. **B.** Tibialis posterior
    C. Posterior tibial artery
58. **A.** Medial part of anterior intercondylar area
59. **C.** Lateral pterygoid
60. **C.** Symphysis
61. **D.** Cruciate ligaments
62. **B.** L_1
63. **A.** Optic nerve
64. **B.** Musculocutaneous nerve
65. **C.** Long thoracic nerve
66. **C.** Posterolateral sapce
67. **D.** Lacunar ligament
68. **A.** Stylopharyngeus
69. **B.** Middle meningeal artery
70. **B.** Right umbilical vein
71. **B.** Medial geniculate body
72. **C.** Flexion at MP and extension at IP joint
73. **C.** S_2 S_3 S_4
74. **A.** Nucleus tractus solitarius
75. **C.** Dorsal scapular
76. **C.** First lumbar
77. **D.** Ovary

78. **A.** Crossed anteriorly by gonadal artery
79. **A.** Spinal cord
80. **B.** Sublingual gland
81. **C.** 8 weeks
82. **C.** Bulbospongiosus muscle
83. **D.** Tail of pancreas
84. **C.** Oligodendroglia
85. **D.** Fasciculus gracilis
86. **A.** Abduction
    B. Intorsion
    D. Depression
87. **A.** Brachialis
    B. Biceps
    C. Brachioradialis
88. **D.** Dentate nuclei
89. **C.** Prepatellar
90. **A.** Median
91. **C.** $C_{5, 6, 7}$ (Root value of radial nv. is C_5 to T_1)
92. **A.** L_3
93. **A.** C_5-C_6
94. **A.** CBD, Hepatic artery, Portal vein
95. **D.** Superior gluteal nerve
96. **D.** Ulnar nerve
97. **C.** 31
98. **D.** S_2 S_3 S_4
99. **C.** C_3 C_4 C_5
100. **C.** Clavicle
101. **D.** Sigmoid sinus and straight sinus
102. **B.** 22
103. **C.** Arch of aorta
104. **A.** Stylo pharyngeus
105. **C.** Inferior vena cava
106. **A.** Flexion
107. **D.** Adductor brevis
108. **A.** 2nd to 4th [Ref. BDC-III-136]
109. **B.** Sensory branches
110. **B.** Serratus anterior [Ref. BDC-I-40]
111. **D.** Dorsiflexion [Ref. Snell-619,568]
112. **B.** Gluteus medius
     D. Gluteus minimus
113. **D.** Capitate
114. **B.** Nucleus ambiguous

2 *Biochemistry*

I. PROTEINS AND AMINO ACIDS

1. Transmembrane Proteins (Integral proteins): Properties [Harper 26th/P-450]

"SAGA"

Span the lipid bilayer
Amphiphatic in nature
Globular proteins
Asymmetrical distribution.

☑ The hydrophilic amino acids in the transmembrane proteins are located at the ends while the hydrophobic amino acids lie within the core.

2. Essential Amino Acids Lippincot Fig.20.2]

<**PVT. TIM HALL** always argues, never tires >
Phenylalanine, **V**aline, **T**hreonine
Tryptophan, **I**soleucine, **M**ethionine
Histidine, **A**rginine, **L**eucine, **L**ysine
"Always argues": the A is for Arg, not Asp.
"Never tires": T is not Tyrosine, but is both Thr and Trp.

☑ Also: Histidine and Arginine are semiessential amino acids.

Mnemonic : <**His Arg**uments are not so essential.>
Another good mnemonic is:
<**A**ny **H**elp **I**n **L**earning **T**hese **L**ittle **M**olecules **P**roves **Tr**uly **V**aluable! >
Arginine, **H**istidine, **I**soleucine, **L**eucine,
Threonine, **L**ysine, **M**ethionine,
Phenylalanine, **Tr**yptophan, **V**aline

3. <u>Amino Acids</u>: <u>Classification based on Structure</u> [Harper 26th Ed/P-16]

"**OH**! **S**he **T**ried **T**hrice, **B**ut **H**e **L**iked **A**rchie, **S**o **C**atharine **M**ust **S**uffer"

Amino acids containing side chain with–OH group:

OH-OH containing AA
S-Serine
T-Tyrosine
T-Threonine

Basic amino acids:

B-Basic amino acids
H-Histidine
L-Lysine
A-Arginine

Sulphur containing amino acids:

S-Sulphur containing AA
C-Cystine
M-Methionine
S-Sulphur containing AA.

4. <u>Amino Acid Containing Imino Group</u>:

<I'm A Pro>

<u>**Im**</u>ino <u>**A**</u>cid group is present in <u>**Pro**</u>line.

5. <u>Aromatic amino acids:</u>

<HTTP://Aromatic.com>

Histidine
Tryptophan
Tyrosine
Phenylalanine

☑ Aromatic amino acids can absorb UV light of wavelength 240 nm.

6. Indole Ring is Present in Tryptophan:

<**Ind**ian **Fan**

Indole = Trypto**phan**

7. There are 2 Amino Acids with Acidic Side Chains:

Glutamic acid (Glutamate)
Aspartic acid (Aspartate)

8. Basic Side Chains

<**Basic**ally, **hist**ories **are** **l**ies>
The **Basic** amino acids are **hist**idine, **ar**ginine, and **l**ysine.

9. Hydrophobic Amino Acids [Lippincot-2]

<**P**apa **GAV** **Me** **T**en **PIL**s without water !>
Proline
Glycine
Alanine
Valine
Methionine
Tryptophan (it is a **10** letter word)
Phenylalanine
Isoleucine
Leucine
Without water—to remember that they are hydrophobic.

10. Amino Acids Arrangement in a Polypeptide [Lippincot 3rd/P-14]

<AmiNo aCids go from **N**-terminal to **C**-terminal>
All amino acid sequences are read from the N- to the C- terminal end of the peptide (from NH_2~ terminal to COO~ terminal).

11. Amino acids producing Succniyl CoA: [Harper 25th Ed/P-339]

<**I'M** **V**ery **T**ired, **S**ir>
I- Isoleucine
M- Methionine
V- Valine
T- Threonine
S- Succniyl CoA
Alternatively: <Success Is Most Vital Today>

12. Branched-Chain Amino Acids used by Skeletal Muscles in Fasting State [Lippincot-3rd P-264]

<**M**uscles **LIVe** in **Mapels**>
Leucine
Isoleucine
Valine

☑ These branch-chained amino acids are primarily metabolized in skeletal muscles rather than liver.

☑ An inherited deficiency of *branched-chain á-ketoacid dehydrogenase* results in the accumulation of the branched chain keto acid substrates in the urine causing a sweet odour in the urine. This is known as **Maple Syrup urine disease**. (*Think of cutting branches of a Maple tree.*). Causes severe CNS defects, mental retardation, and death.

13. Catabolism Steps of Branched Chain Amino Acids [Harper 25th Ed/P-340]

<**Tr**uck hit the **Ox** to **De**ath>:
-**Tr**ansamination
-**Ox**idative decarboxylation
-**De**hydrogenation

14. Urea Cycle [Lippincot 2nd /P-237]

<**O**rdinary, **C**areless **C**ramming **A**s **A** **F**ool is **A**ctually **U**seless>
Ornithine
Carbamoyl phosphate
Citrulline
Aspartate
Aginosuccinate
Fumarate
Arginine
Urea.

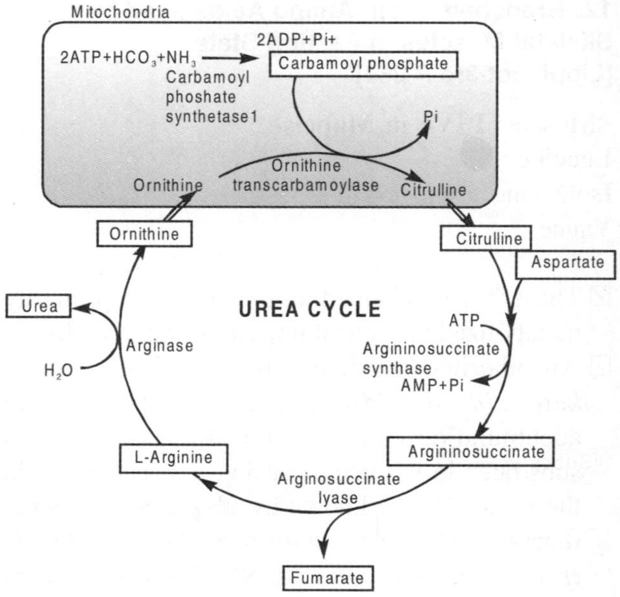

Fig. 2.1

Note:

☑ 2 products go in the cycle: **C**arbamoyl phosphate and **A**spartate

☑ 2 products go out of the cycle: **F**umarate and **U**rea

☑ 4 products remain in the cycle: **O**rnithine, **C**itrulline, **A**ginosuccinate and **A**rginine

15. Methionine Metabolism: [Lippincot 3rd Ed/P-262]

<**Homo-cysteine** can either **Succ**essfully make **Cysteine** or go **home** to **Meet SAM**.>
See Fig. 2.2.

Go home – go to the starting point
Meet – **Met**hionine
SAM – **S**-**a**denosyl**m**ethionine
Successfully – **Succ**inyl CoA
THF = Tetrahydrofolate

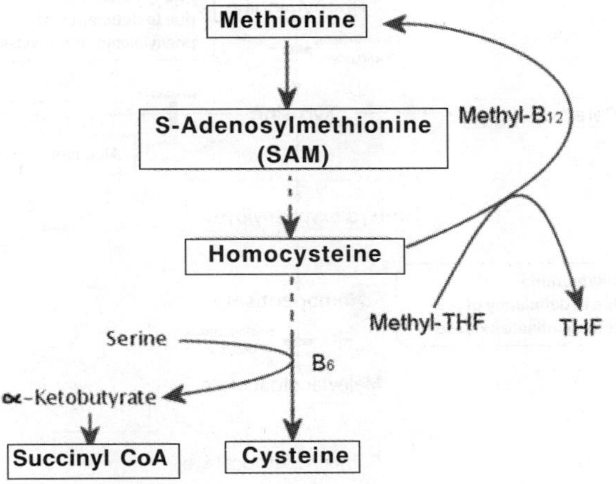

Fig. 2.2: Methionine metabolism (simplified)

Also know:

☑ SAM is a high-energy compound, which does not have phosphate.

☑ SAM is the principal source of methyl in our body.

☑ Since cysteine can be generated in the body from methionine, it is not an essential amino acid.

☑ Homicysteine is an important risk factor for coronary heart disease and Vit. B_6, B_{12}, and foliate help in reducing its level in blood.

16. Phenylketonuria and Alkaptonuria [Lippincot 3rd Ed/P-267]

<PPT. of HAM>

Phenylketonuria occurs between **P**henylalanine and **T**yrosine.

Alkaptonuria occurs between **H**omogentisate and **M**aleylacetoacetate.

See Fig. 2.3 on next page.

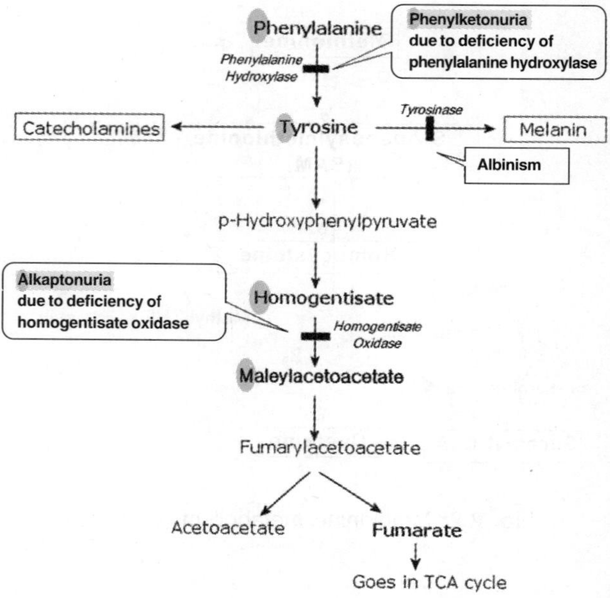

Fig. 2.3: Phenylalanine metabolism

17. Phenylketonuria: Which Enzyme is Deficient [Lippincot/P-268]

PHenylketonuria is caused by a deficiency of: **P**henylalanine **H**ydroxylase.

Phenylalanine Hydroxylase

Phenylalanine ⟶ Tyrosine

18. Phenylketonuria Findings [Harrison-2332]

<Phenyl-Keton-Uria = PKU>
Pale hair and skin
Krazy (Seizures, Severe mental retardation)
Unpleasant smell (mo**U**sy odour)

19. Catecholamines Synthesis:

<**P**harmacists **T**ry *To* **D**ope **D**rugs *Causing* **N**egative **E**ffects.>
See Fig. 2.4

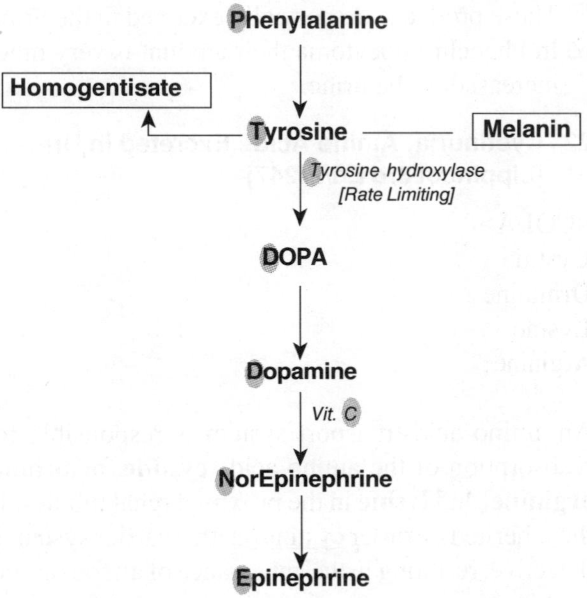

Fig. 2.4: Synthesis of catecholamines

20. Tryptophan vs. Tyrosine: [Lippincot 2nd P-266,267]

Tyro**sine**—Think of a **sin** and it will raise your adrena**line.**
Trypto**phan**—Makes **Fan**tasies by raising **serotonin** in the brain.

☑ Tyrosine makes adrenaline and tryptophan makes serotonin.

21. Vanillyl Mandelic Acid: [Lippincot 2nd Ed/P-267]

<VMA>
VMA and **M**etanephrine are formed from **A**drenaline.

Also know:
☑ VMA and Normetanephrine are formed from Noradrenaline.

☑ These products are normally excreted in the urine.
☑ In Pheochromocytoma their amount is very much increased in the urine.

22. Cystinuria: Amino Acids Excreted in Urine [Lippincot 3rd Ed/P-247]

<COLA>
Cystine
Ornithine
Lysine
Arginine

An amino acid transport system is responsible for reabsorption of the amino acids **cystine**, **ornithine**, **arginine**, and **lysine** in the proximal renal tubules. In the inherited disorder cystinuria, this carrier system is defective, resulting in the appearance of all four amino acids in the urine. Cystinuria occurs at a frequency of 1 in 7000 individuals, ranking it one of the most common inherited diseases, and the most common genetic error of amino acid transport. The disease expresses itself clinically by the precipitation of cystine to form kidney stones (calculi), which can block the urinary tract. Oral hydration is an important part of treatment for this disorder.

II. CARBOHYDRATES

1. Glycogen Storage Diseases

a. Glycogen Storage: Names of Types I through VI [H-2321]

<Viagra **P**ills **C**ause **A**bsolute **M**ale **H**ardness>

Type I	Von Gierke's
Type II	Pompe's
Type III	Cori's
Type IV	Anderson's
Type V	McArdle's
Type VI	Her's

b. Type 1 Glycogen Storage Disease [H-2321]

Type 1 = one (Von)
Von Gierke's disease

Remember:
< **KIL Von**>
- Affects liver, **Kidney** & **Intestines**:
- Fatty **Liver**, hepatomegaly
- Muscles are not involved

a. Pompe's Disease: [Lippincot-3rd-128]

<In **Pompe**'s disease there is defect in the **Pump** of heart.>
- Patient dies early by heart failure.
- There is massive cardiomegaly
- There is deficiency of lysosomal *á-glusosidase* enzyme

b. Anderson's (IV) vs. Cori's (III) enzyme defect [H-2321] [Lippincot 3rd/P-128]

<ABCD>
Anderson's = **B**ranching enzyme defect.
Cori's = **D**ebranching enzyme defect.

☑ *Otherwise, one can't really distinguish between the two clinically.*

c. McArdle's disease: [Lippincot-3rd-128]

<McArdle's disease is a disease of **M**'s>
- **M**uscle glycogen phosphorylase deficient
- **M**uscle cramps
- **M**yoglobinuria with exercise
- **M**ental development is normal

2. Confused with Glycogenesis and Glycogenolysis ?

Look carefully at the last few letters in each word… Glycogenesis contains '-genesis' which means 'make', so it makes glycogen form glucose. Glycogenolysis contains '-lysis' which means 'to break down', so it breaks down glycogen to give glucose and glucose-1-phosphate.

3. Glycolysis [L-94-120]

<**G**oodness **G**racious, **F**ather **F**ranklin **D**id **G**o **B**y **P**icking **P**umpkins **2**(to) **P**repare **P**ies>
See next page for Fig 2.5.

'Did', 'By' and 'Pies' tell you the first part of those three: di-, bi-, and py-.

'PrEPare' tells location of PEP in the process.
Remember irreversible steps by:

Goodness Gracious = Glucokinase

Father **F**ran**K**lin = **F**ospho**F**ructo**K**inase

Pies once **p**repared, cannot be reversed (**P**yruvate kinase)

Also remember the no. of ATP produced:
< 2 × 2 × 2 = 8 >

☑ Total in Anaerobic Glycolysis = **2**ATP
☑ Total in Aerobic Glycolysis= **2**ATP + **2**NADH = **8** ATP
☑ 1 NADH = 3 ATP
☑ Total no. of ATP used up in glycolysis = 2 ATP

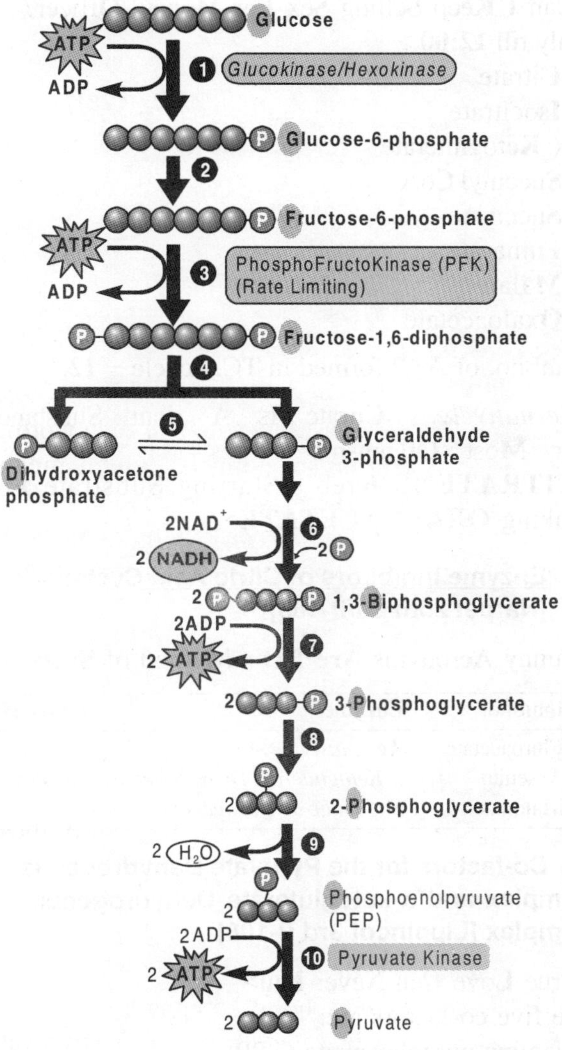

Fig. 2.5: Glycolysis

4. Glucagon Function: [Lippincot 3rd Ed/P-312]

<Mr. **Gluca** has **Gone** to the **cAMP** to bring out some **Glucose**>:

Glucagon elevates glucose by activating cAMP in the hepatocytes.

5 <u>Citric Acid Cycle</u>
[Lippincot P-107] [Harper 25th P-185]

<**C**an **I** **K**eep **S**elling **S**ex **F**or **M**oney, **O**fficer? … Only till **12:00** >

1. **C**itrate
2. **I**socitrate
3. ⟨ **K**etogluterate
4. **S**uccinyl CoA
5. **S**uccinate
6. **F**umarate
7. **M**alate
8. **O**xaloacetate

Total no. of ATP formed in TCA cycle = **12**.

Alternatively: <**C**itrate **I**s **A** **S**our **S**ubstance **F**or **M**ost **O**rganisms>
<**CITRATE IS** **K**reb's **S**tarting **S**ubstrate **F**or **M**aking **OXALOACETATE**>

6. Enzyme Inhibitors of Citric Acid Cycle: [Harper 25th Ed/P-185]

<**F**unny **Ac**ronyms **Ar**e **KD**'s **M**ethod of **Succ**ess>

	Inhibitor	Enzyme
1	**F**luroacetate	***Ac**onitase*
2	**Ar**senite	*á-**K**etogluterate **D**ehydrogenase complex*
3	**M**alonate	***Succ**inate dehydrogenase*

7. Co-factors for the Pyruvate Dehydrogenase Complex and α-ketoglutarate Dehydrogenase Complex [Lippincot 3rd P-108]

<**T**rue **L**ove **C**an **N**ever **F**ail>
The five co-factors are:
Thiamine pyrophosphate (TPP)
Lipoic acid
CoA
NAD
FAD

☑ The pyruvate dehydrogenase complex converts pyruvate to acetyl CoA in the mitochondria.

☑ The α-ketoglutarate dehydrogenase enzyme converts α-ketoglutarate to succinyl CoA in the TCA cycle.

III. NUCLEIC ACIDS, PURINES AND PYRIMIDINES

1. Purines vs. Pyramidines

Pyrimidines are "**CUT**" from purines.

☑ Pyrimidines are **C**ytosine, **U**racil, **T**hiamine and are one ring structures.

☑ Purines are double ring structures.

2. DNA Bond Strength (Chargaff's Rule) [Lippincot-395]

<Crazy Glue>
<Char = Gaff's rule>

☑ There are 3 bonds between Cytosine and Guanine (G=C) (stronger bonds like Crazy Glue).

☑ Whereas the (A=T) only have 2 H-bonds (weaker bonds).

This is relevant to DNA replication, as the weaker A=T will be the site where RNA primer makes the initial break.

Also know:

☑ DNA that contains more G=C will have higher melting point, as more energy will be required to break them.

☑ The temperature at which one half of helical structure is lost is known as **melting temperature.**

2. DNA Structure [Lippincot P-344]

<Nucleo**side** is only a **side** of Nucleotide>
Nucleotide = Base + Sugar + Phosphate
Nucleoside = Base + Sugar

Example:
Base = Adenine
Nucleoside = Adenosine
Nucleotide = AMP
Sugar = Ribose in RNA and Deoxyribose in DNA

4. Post Translational Modifications of Eukaryotic mRNA: [Harper 25th P-448, Lippincot P-385]

<Just after the birth of RNA we have to do it's **CPR**>
The primary transcripts are extensively modified in the nucleus after transcription.
These modifications usually include:
5' **C**apping
3' **P**olyadenylation
Removal of introns
☑ Vit. K and Vit. C are important in post translation modification

5. Exon vs. Intron Function [Lippincot P-386]

<**E**xons are **E**xpressed>
<**I**n**T**rons are left **I**n **T**rash>

6. Function of Southern vs. Northern vs. Western blots

<**SN0W DR0P**>
Match up the 1st word letter with 2nd word letter:

Southern=**D**NA
Northern=**R**NA
Western=**P**rotein
(The 0's in snowdrop are zeros, since there is no Eastern blot.)

7. RNA and DNA Polymerase [Lippincot 2nd P-374]

DNA polymerase – **D**oes **N**eed **A** **P**rimer
RNA polymerase – **R**equires **N**o **P**rimer

8. RNA Polymerases [Lippincot 3rd P-421, 414]

<**1,2,3** = **RMT** (in Rhythm)>
☑ RNA Polymerase **I** makes **r**RNA (**R**ampant - the most abundant type of RNA)
☑ RNA Polymerase **II** makes **m**RNA (**M**assive - the largest type of RNA)

☑ RNA Polymerase **III** makes **t**RNA (**T**iny - the smallest type of RNA and T shaped)

9. Eukaryote Polymerases: [Harper 25th P-424]

Alpha—L**A**gging strand synthesis
Delta—Lea**D**ing strand synthesis
Ga**M**ma- **M**itochondrial DNA synthesis
Beta and Epsilon involved in DNA repair

10. Structural forms of DNA [Lippincot 2nd - 360]

<**BAZ**>
B-Form—10 Base pairs per 360°—Right handed—Most common
A-Form—11 Base pairs per 360°—Right handed—Moderately dehydrated B-form
Z-Form—12 Base pairs per 360°—Left handed—Zigzag form

11. DNA Topoisomerase: [Lippincot 2nd – 365]

Type-**I** DNA topoisomerase – Cut only **1** strand of DNA double helix.
Type-**II** DNA topoisomerase – Cuts **both** strands of DNA.

☑ DNA topoisomerases are enzymes responsible for providing a mechanism for removing supercoils during DNA replication.

12. DNA Helicase [Lippincot-364]

DNA Helicase are enzymes which disrupt the **DNA Helix** and cause it's unwinding.

13. Protein Synthesis: Initiation and Stop Codons [Lippincot 3rd/P-436]

☑ Initiation codon:
<**AUG** → **Aug**ments protein synthesis>
AUG is the initiating codon and it codes for methionine.

☑ Stop codons:
UGA —**U** **G**o **A**way
UAA —**U** **A**re **A**way
UAG —**U** **A**re **G**one

14. Protein synthesis : Energy required [Lippincot 3rd/P-434]

<**ATP** in tRNA **A**ctivation >
<**GTP** in tRNA **G**ripping and **G**oing places >

☑ Cleavage of 4 high-energy bonds is required for the addition of one amino acid to the growing polypeptide chain.

☑ 2 energy comes from conversion of ATP to AMP + 2Pi in tRNA Activation by *aminoacyl-tRNA synthase*.

☑ 1 energy comes from GTP used in binding of aminoacyl-tRNA to the A-site (tRNA **G**ripping).

☑ 1 energy comes from GTP used in translocation step (**G**oing places).

Also know:

Mnemonic: <*Amino-Acyl tRNA Synthase* = Always Acts Totally Safe>

☑ A specific *aminoacyl-tRNA synthase* is present for each type of amino acid which binds to a specific amino acid.

☑ This reaction is so specific that *aminoacyl-tRNA synthase* is called as the "Fidelity enzyme".

15. DNA Binding Motifs in Transcription Factors: [Harper 25th-480][Ganong 22nd -23]

Several motifs mediate the binding of regulatory proteins to DNA:

<**Unzip Lucy** with your **Zealous Fingers** and take **Turns** to **Look** inside>

- **Leucine zipper**
- **Zinc finger** (commonest)
- helix-**Turn**-helix
- helix-**Loop**-helix

☑ Over 80% of known transcription factors have one of four DNA-bonding motifs.

☑ The protein- DNA interactions are maintained by hydrogen bonds and Van-der-Waals forces.

16. Mitochondrial DNA (mt DNA) Properties [Ganong 22nd P-836,837]

<mt DNA>

mt stands for:

Maternal **T**ransfer

Mutates **T**remendously (high mutation rate)

Most sequences are **T**ranslated

17. Mitochondrial diseases: Important ones [H-16th Ed/P-2535] [Harper 25th Ed/P838]

<Ragged Labourer Kissed My Melenas>

Alternatively: **<13 Labourers Kiss My Red Melenas>**

- **Ragged** red fibers (histological feature)
- **Leber** Hereditary Optic Neuropathy (LHON) – No myopathy and ragged red fibers
- **KSS** - Kearns-Sayre Syndrome
- **My**oclonus Epilepsy with Ragged Red Fibers (MERRF)
- **MELAS** –Mitochondrial Encephalopathy with Lactic Acidosis and Stroke like episodes

☑ The mitochondrial DNA encodes for **13** protein subunits of the respiratory chain.

18. Purine Metabolism and Salvage: [Lippincot 3rd P-294] [H 16th -2312]

Lesch-Nyhan syndrome and Kelly-Seegmiller syndrome:

Hypoxanthine and guanine are two intermediates formed during the breakdown of purine nucleotides (AMP and GMP). These two intermediates will eventually form uric acid if they remain unused which is excreted as waste. However, in our body it is possible to conserve these two products by an enzyme

Hypoxanthine-guanine phosphoribosyl-transferase (HPRT). This enzyme can convert hypoxanthine to IMP and guanine to GMP which are reutilized to form purine nucleotides and DNA. This pathway is called 'Salvage Pathway of Purines' (see Fig.2.6)

In Lesch-Nyhan syndrome there is virtually complete deficiency of HPRT. This deficiency results in inability to salvage hypoxanthine and guanine, from which excessive amounts of uric acid are produced. It is an X-linked recessive disease. Clinical presentation is that of a severe form of gout. In addition, characteristic neurological features of the disorder include self-mutilation and involuntary movements mental retardation choreoathetosis.

☑ Remember a generalized rule: "X-linked recessive diseases are always severe."

In Kelly-Seegmiller syndrome there is a partial deficiency of HPRT and it is associated with hyperuricemia but no CNS manifestation.

Mnemonics:

<**L**esch-**N**yhan **S**yndrome = **L**acks **N**ucleotides **S**alvages (of purine)>

<**K**elly-**S**eegmiller **S**yndrome = **K**eeps **S**ome **S**alvage>

HPRT → <**H**as **P**urine **R**eutilizing **T**echinique.>

Note: Some books mention HPRT as HGPRT. Change the above mnemonic to

<**H**as **G**ot **P**urine **R**eutilizing **T**echinique>

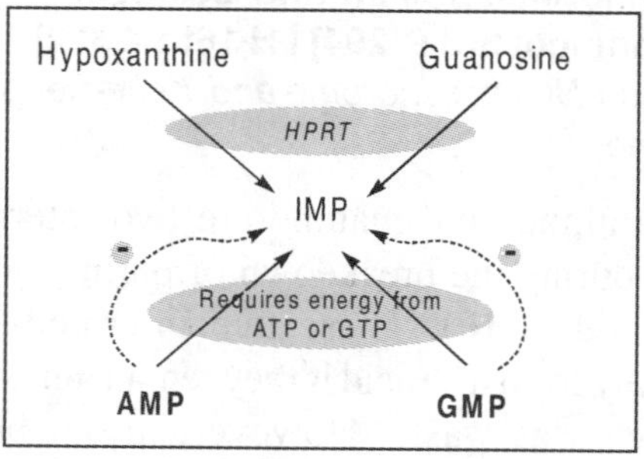

Fig. 2.6

19. Adenosine Deaminase Deficiency (ADD) and Severe Combined Immunodeficiency Disease (SCID) [Lippincot 3rd/P-299]

<s**CID** happens to **KID**s>
<For those with **SCID**, problems **ADD** up quickly>

- Severe **A**denosine **D**eaminase **D**eficiency (**ADD**) can cause **SCID**.
- In ADD, excess dATP is formed which inhibits *ribonucleotide reductase*.
- *ribonucleotide reductase* is required to convert ribose to deoxyribose. It's inhibition prevents DNA synthesis and thus lowers lymphocyte count.
- This disease occurs in children and they die by 2 years of age.
- SCID was the first disease to be treated by experimental human gene therapy.

☑ SCID = Severe Combined Immunodeficiency Disease (both T& B cell deficiency).
(See Fig. 2.7 in Purine degradation and salvage)

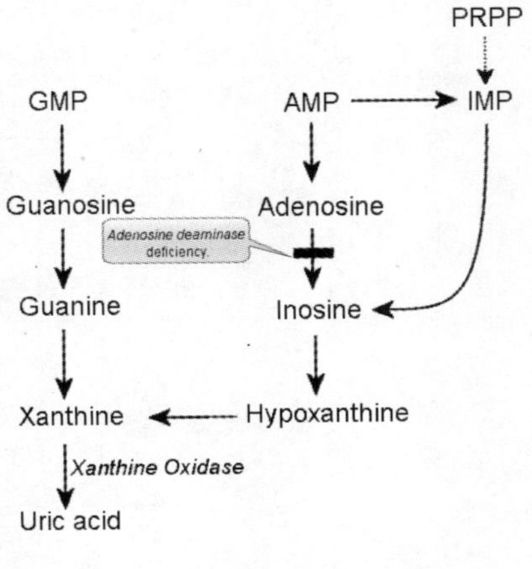

Fig. 2.7: Degradation of purine

20. <u>MycoPhenolic Acid: Function</u> [Lippincot 3rd -293]

<**IMP** dehydrogenase is **I**nhibited by **M**yco**P**henolate.>

- Mycophenolic acid is a reversible, non-competative inhibitor of Inosine monophosphate dehydrogenase.
- *IMP dehydrogenase* is required in conversion of IMP to Xanthosine monophosphate (XMP) which is then converted to GMP.
- This drug is used to prevent <u>graft rejection</u>.

$$\text{IMP} \xrightarrow{\textit{IMP dehydrogenase}} \text{XMP} \longrightarrow \text{GMP}$$

IV. LIPIDS

1. Unsaturated Fatty Acid [Lippincot-173]

"O' LiLi Are U Nervous ?"
Oleic acid
Linoleic acid
Linolenic acid
Arachidonic acid
Unsaturated fatty acids
Nervonic acid

2. Fatty Acids: Number of Unsaturated (Double) Bonds [Lippincot-173]

Fatty acid	*Structure*	*No. of double bonds*
Oleic acid	18:1(9)	1
Linoleic acid	18:2(9,12)	2
Linolenic acid	18:3(9,12,15)	3
Arachidonic acid	20:4(5,8,11,14)	4

☑ Longer the name, more the number of unsaturated bonds. Also it fits perfectly in the above mnemonic.

3. Ketone as Fuel in Fasting State [Shindey Chatterjee]

"In fasting state two organs which must **ket-on (keep-on)** are **Brain** and **Heart**."

On prolonged starvation, brain and heart cells can adopt to using ketone bodies as a major source of energy. The liver is the chief organ which makes ketones. However liver cannot utilize ketone bodies as fuel.

4. β-oxidation: End Product [Harper-25th/P-240]

☑ β-oxidation of even chain fatty acids produces even numbered carbon residue–Acetyl CoA (2-carbons).

☑ β-oxidation of odd chain fatty acids produces odd numbered carbon residue—Propionyl CoA (3-carbons).

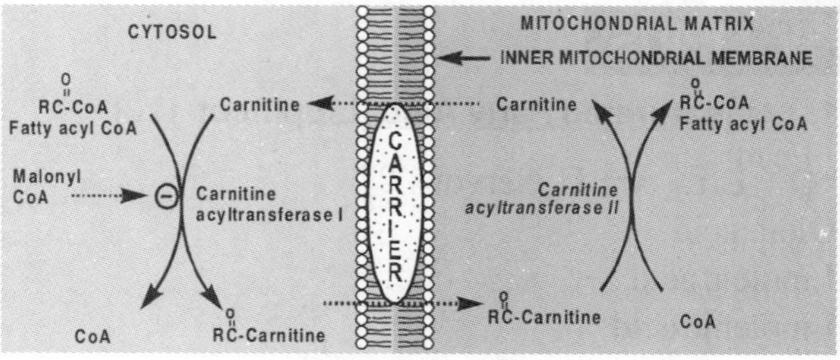

Fig. 2.8: Carnitine shuttle

5. <u>Carnitine Shuttle</u> [Lippincot 2nd—182, Fig. 2.8]

<Fatty acids need a special **'Car'** for their transport from cytosol to mitochondria for beta oxidation>

This special 'Car' is **Car**nitine and the process is called Carnitine shuttle.

Malonyl CoA causes malfunction in this Car ® It inhibits Carnitine acyltransferase I.

6. <u>Sphingolipidoses: (Lysosomal storage diseases)</u> [Lippincot-3rd–208] [H-16th -2316]

In a normal individual, synthesis and degradation of sphingolipids are balanced, so that the amount of these compounds present in membranes is constant. If a specific hydrolase required for the degradation process is partially or totally missing, a sphingolipid accumulates in the lysosomes. Lipid storage diseases caused by these deficiencies are called sphingolipidoses.

The important ones are listed below:

<u>Fabry's disease</u> :

<Burning and Galloping in seX Fever>

- Burning—Burning pain in lower extremities
- Reddish purple skin rash (as if burned)
- **a Gal**loping—α-**Gal**actosidase A deficiency
- se**X**—**X**-linked recessive
- Fever—Fabry.

Another good mnemonic is:

< OH! FABRY'S >

Opacities in cornea and lens
Heart failure
Foam cells found in glomeruli and tubules/febrile episodes
Alpha galactosidase A deficiency/Angiokeratomas/ Acroparesthesia
Burning pain in extremities
Renal failure
YX genotype (Male, X linked recessive)
Sphingolipidoses.

Tay-Sach's disease:
Sandhoff's disease:] <Take Some **Sand** and do **Sizzling** and **Blinding** Magical **Hex**>

- **T**ake Some–Tay-Sach's
- **Sand–Sand**hoff's
- **Sizzling–Seizures**
- **Blinding–Blindness** and cherry red macula
- **M**agical–**M**ental retardation
- **Hex**–β-**Hex**osaminidase deficiency (type A in Tay-Sach's; type A & B in Sandhoff's).

Niemann-Pick disease:

<No Man Picks All his Sphincters>

- **No man picks** - Niemann-Pick
- **All**–All types of manifestations: Neurological, liver and spleen enlargement, skeletal disease (only in type B), macular degeneration, foam cells in bone marrow, pulmonary infilterate.
- **Sphin**cters–**Sphin**gomyelinase deficiency.

Gaucher's disease:

<**Glucher** has a lot of **Common Sense**>

- **Glu-cher**—Gaucher disease and **'Glu-'** for β-**Glu**cosidase.
- **Common**—Most common lysosomal storage disease.
- **Sense**—Sense is preserved (i.e. CNS involvement is rare in type 1).

7. Alphabetical List of Lysosomal Storage Diseases

Activator Deficiency/GM2 Gangliosidosis
Alpha-Mannosidosis
Aspartylglucosaminuria

Cholesteryl ester storage disease
Chronic Hexosaminidase A Deficiency
Cystinosis
Danon disease
Fabry disease
Farber Disease
Fucosidosis
Galactosialidosis
Gaucher Disease
- Type I
- Type II
- Type III

GM1 Gangliosidosis
- Infantile
- Late infantile/Juvenile
- Adult/Chronic

I-Cell disease/Mucolipidosis II
Infantile Free Sialic Acid Storage Disease/ISSD
Juvenile Hexosaminidase A Deficiency
Krabbe Disease
- Infantile Onset
- Late Onset

Metachromatic Leukodystrophy
Mucopolysaccharidoses disorders
- Pseudo-Hurler polydystrophy/Mucolipidosis IIIA
- MPSI Hurler Syndrome
- MPSI Scheie Syndrome
- MPS I Hurler-Scheie Syndrome
- MPS II Hunter syndrome
- Sanfilippo Type A/MPS III A
- Sanfilippo Type B/MPS III B
- Sanfilippo Type C/MPS III C
- Sanfilippo Type D/MPS III D
- Morquio Type A/MPS IVA
- Morquio Type B/MPS IVB
- MPS IX Hyaluronidase Deficiency
- MPS VI Maroteaux-Lamy
- MPS VII Sly Syndrome
- Mucolipidosis I/ Sialidosis

- Mucolipidosis IIIC
- Mucolipidosis IV

Multiple sulfatase deficiency
Niemann-Pick Disease

- Type A
- Type B
- Type C

Neuronal Ceroid Lipofuscinoses

- CLN6 Disease - Atypical Late Infantile
- CLN6 Disease - Late Onset variant
- CLN6 Disease - Early Juvenile
- Batten-Spielmeyer-Vogt/Juvenile NCL/CLN3 disease
- Finnish Variant Late Infantile CLN5
- Jansky-Bielschowsky/Late infantile CLN2/ TPP1 Disease
- Kufs/Adult-onset NCL/CLN4 disease
- Northern Epilepsy/variant late infantile CLN8
- Santavuori-Haltia/Infantile CLN1/PPT disease
- Beta-Mannosidosis

Pompe disease/Glycogen storage disease II
Pycnodysostosis
Sandhoff Disease/Adult Onset/GM2 Gangliosidosis
Sandhoff Disease/GM2 Gangliosidosis - Infantile
Sandhoff Disease/GM2 gangliosidosis - Juvenile
Schindler disease
Salla disease/Sialic Acid Storage Disease
Tay-Sachs/GM2 gangliosidosis
Wolman Disease

V. MISCELLANEOUS

1. Hypervitaminosis A: Signs and Symptoms [Ghai 121, H-408]

<Increased Vitamin A makes you **HARD**>
Headache/ Hepatomegaly
Anorexia/ Alopecia
Really painful bones
Dry skin/ Drowsiness

☑ Hypervitaminosis A causes raised Intracranial tension – (Pseudotumor cerebri)
☑ Carotinoids do not cause toxicity except yellow colour of skin.

2. Vitamin B5 (Niacin, Nicotinic acid) Deficiency: Pellagra Syndrome [Ghai-125, H-405]

<The **4 D**'s of pellagra>
Dermatitis
Diarrhea
Dementia
Death

☑ Niacin can be formed in the body by conversion of L-Tryptophan to niacin.
☑ However deficiency can occur in maize eaters due to high leucin content which interferes with above reaction.
☑ Other causes of deficiency: Hartnup disease, Carcinoid syndrome, Alcoholism.
☑ Characteristic skin rash—Casal's necklace

Remember:
<CATCH Me>
Casal's necklace
Alcoholism
Tryptophan conversion defect
Carcinoid syndrome

Hartnup disease
Maize eaters

3. <u>Van den Bergh Reaction</u> (Jaundice Test)

<<u>I</u>ndirect bilirubin = <u>U</u>nconjugated bilirubin>
Both start with vowels (a, e, i, o, u) so they go together: Indirect and Unconjugated.
Therefore Direct bilirubin is conjugated bilirubin.

4. <u>Inherited Hyperbilirubinemia: Conjugated & Unconjugated</u>

<Use **CNG**>
Unconjugated = **C**riggler **N**azar Syndrome & **G**ilbert Syndrome

<**CD Rom**>
Conjugated = **D**ubin-Johnson and **R**otor Syndrome

<u>5.</u> Sickle Cell Disease Pathophysiology [Lippincot P-36]

SICKle cell disease is due to a Substitution of the SICKsth (6th) amino acid of the B chain.
(Glutamate is replaced by Valine)

6. <u>Adrenaline mechanism at β-receptors</u> [KDT/P-111]

<**ABC** of Adrenaline>
Adrenaline—> activates **B**eta receptors—> increases **C**yclic AMP

7. Diatery Fibers: [Harper 24th/P-628]

<**PMCH L**acks **PG**'s >

1. **P**ectins
2. **M**ucilage
3. **C**ellulose
4. **H**emicellulose
5. **L**ignin
6. **P**entosans
7. **G**ums

8. Electron Transport Chain Target: Inhibitors [Lippincot P-76 , Harrison/P-128]

Roten**one** is a site specific inhibitor of Site **one**.
Dimercaprol inhibits site **2**
Carbon monoxide (**CO**) blocks Cytochrome Oxidase (**CO**) - Site 3

☑ *Others are:*
Site 1 inhibitors – Barbiturates, Rotenone
Site 2 inhibitors – Antimycin, Dimercaprol (BAL)
Site 3 inhibitors – Cyanide, H_2S, CO

9. Enzymes: Classification [Lippincot/P-53]

<Over The HILL>
Oxidoreductases
Transferases
Hydrolases
Isomerases
Ligases
Lyases

☑ Enzymes get reaction over the hill.
See Fig. 2.9

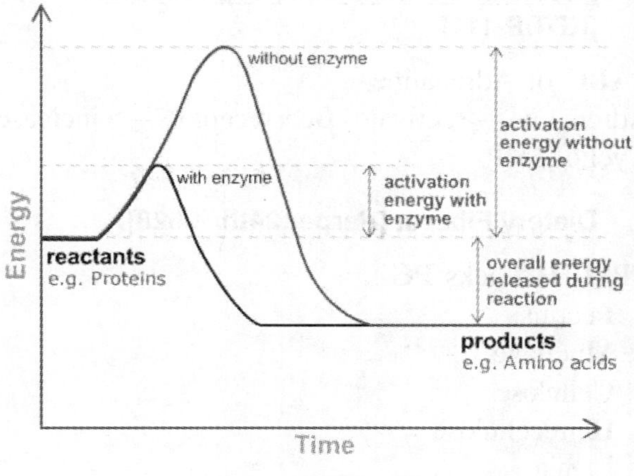

Fig. 2.9

10. <u>Enzyme Kinetics: Competitive vs. Non-Competitive Inhibition</u> [Lippincot P-60]

With **K**ompetitive inhibition: **K**m increases; no change in V_{max}
With **N**on-kompetitive inhibition: **N**o change in Km; V_{max} decreases.

☑ Km = Substrate concentration at which reaction velocity is ½ V_{max}
☑ Vmax = Maximum velocity of reaction

See Fig. 2.10

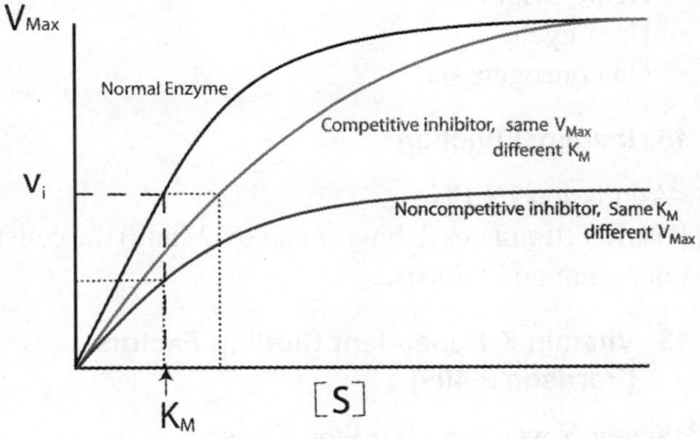

Fig. 2.10

11. Cation vs. Anion: Positive vs. Negative

The **'t'** in cation looks like a plus sign: < **ca+ion** >
Cation is positive ion, anion is negative ion.

Cation goes towards the Cathode (negative electrode)
Anion goes towards the Anode (positive electrode)

12. Metabolisms Occurring in Cytoplasm are:

<**S**ome **G**ood **P**eople **H**aving **F**un **T**ogether>
- **S**teroid synthesis
- **G**lycolysis

- **P**rotein synthesis
- **HMP** shunt
- **F**atty acid synthesis
- **T**CA cycle

13. Metabolism in Mitochondria:

<Mity OAK>

Mity – **Mit**ochondria
- β-**O**xidation
- **A**cetyl CoA production
- **K**rebs cycle

14. Metabolism Common to Both Sites:

<Use both arms to HUG>
- **H**eme synthesis
- **U**rea cycle
- **G**luconeogenesis

15. Insulin: Function

<Admission **IN-PG**>

INsulIN stimulates 2 things to go IN 2 (into) the cells: Potassium and Glucose.

16. Vitamin K Dependent Clotting Factors [Harrison P-409]

<Seven Never Tries To Stop Clots>

Clotting Factors :

Seven

Nine

Ten

Two

Protein **S**

Protein **C**.

17. Change in pH at pKa [Harper 25th Ed/P-23]

<At p**K**a … pH is **K**onstant >

At values close to pKa, the buffer solution resists changes in pH most effectively.

18. <u>Collagen Types and Distribution</u>: [Lippincot 3rd -44]

<Collagen types go **from hard to soft** in distribution>
type I = bone, tendons, dentine of teeth, (cornea)
type II = cartilage, (vitreous body)
type III (+type I) = skin, blood vessels, smooth muscles
type IV =basement membrane

☑ Exceptions to this rule is Cornea (Type I collagen) and vitreous body (Type II collagen)
☑ Structures with type III collagen also have type I collagen.

9. <u>Serum Enzymes</u>:

<**A**ll **L**iver **T**roubles>
An increase in the enzyme ALT (alanine aminotransferase) is an indication of possible liver damage.
<**C**ardiac **K**nockout.>
An increase in the enzyme CK (creatine kinase) is an indication of possible myocardial infarction.

20. <u>AST vs. ALT</u> [Harper 25th-83]

If you can't remember whether SGOT stands for AST or ALT then remember that
<Both liver and heart H<u>AS GOT</u> it>.
Therefore, **<u>AST</u> = S<u>GOT</u>.**
Conversely: ALT = SGPT

☑ AST has a diagnostic significance in myocardial infraction and ALT has a diagnostic significance in viral hepatitis.

21. Creatinine Kinase (CK) and Lactate Dehydrogenase (LDH) Isoenzymes: [Lippincot 3rd Ed/P-65] [Harper 25th Ed/P82] [Vasudevan 3rd-47]

CK has 3 types :

Isoenzyme	*Subunits*	*Chiefly found in*
CK1	BB	Brain
CK2	MB	Heart
CK3	M M	Skeletal muscles

<u>Mnemonic:</u>
<Our brain is on top… so CK1 is for brain>
<Heart is in middle … so CK2 is for heart>

LDH has 5 types:

Isoenzyme	*Subunits*	*Chiefly found in*
L1	HHHH	Heart
L2	HHHM	RBC, Heart
L3	HHMM	Brain
L4	HMMM	Liver
L5	MMMM	Skeletal muscles

For LDH the above mnemonic is reversed.
Mnemonic: <For some *Ladies (LDH)* their *heart* is more important their *brains*>

22. Fat Soluble Vitamins:

<**FAKED**>
Fat soluble vitamins are **A**, **K**, **E**, and **D**.

23. <u>Vitamin B-complex: Names</u> [Harper 25th Ed/P-627]

<**T**he **R**hythm **N**early **P**roved **C**ontagious>:
In increasing order:
Thiamine (B1)
Riboflavin (B2)
Niacin (B3)
Pyridoxine (B6)
Cobalamin (B12)

24. <u>Phosphorylation Cascade Activation</u>

<In the **Ph**asted (Fasted) state → **Ph**osphorylate>
Phosphorylation cascade is activated when blood glucose low.

25. Heme Synthesis and Porphyrias: [Lippincot 3rd Ed/P279]

Enzymes:

<**H**eme, **U**ltimately **U**nfinished, **C**reates **P**orphyriogenic **F**ragment>

1. **H**ydroxymethylbilane synthase
2. **U**roporphyrinogen III cosynthase
3. **U**roporphyrinogen decarboxylase
4. **C**oproporphyrinogen oxidase
5. **P**rotoporphyrinogen oxidase
6. **F**errochelatase

Porphyrias:

<**A**ll **C**ongenital **P**orphyrias **H**ave **V**ariable **P**resentation>

1. **A**cute Intermittent Porphyria
2. **C**ongenital erythropoetic Porphyria
3. **P**orphyria Cutanea Tarda
4. **H**ereditary Coprophyria
5. **V**ariegate Porphyria
6. erythropoietic **P**rotoporhyria

See Next page for Fig. 2.11

26. Lead Poisioning:

<*ALA Dehydratase:*(ALAD) rhymes with LEAD >
<*Ferrochelatase:* The poor Fello – Chelates lead instead of iron>
AminoLevolunic Acid Dehydrogenase and Ferrochelatase are inhibited in lead poisioning.

27. Uroporphyrinogen:

<Urine is normally colourless ...so uroporphyrinogen is colourless.>
All other intermediates are coloured.

Also know:

☑ ALA synthase is the rate limiting step and is inhibited by Heme and Hemin.

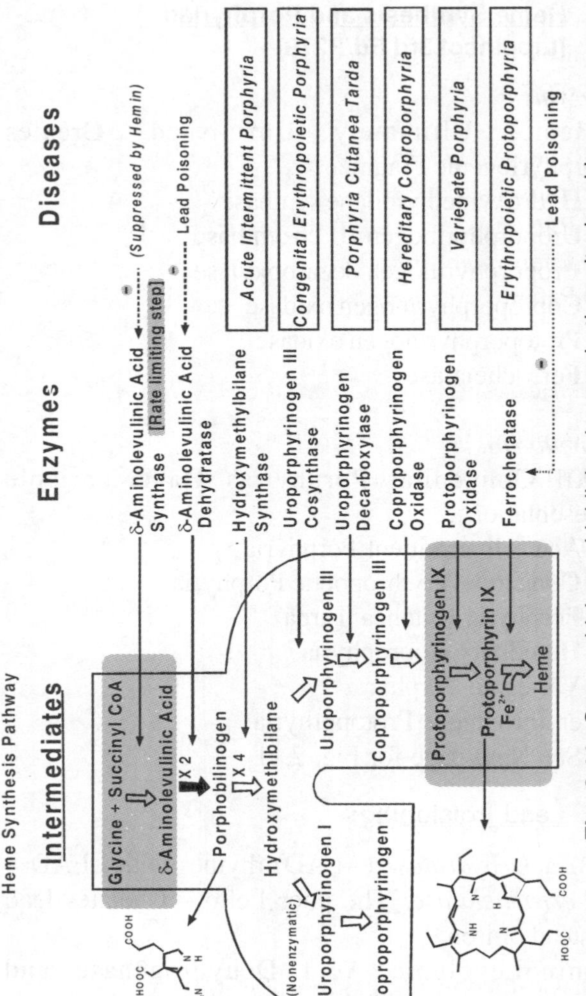

Fig. 2.11: Steps which are highlighted occur in the mitochondria

28. Acute Intermittent Porphyria (AIP) Symptoms [Harrison/P-2305, Lippincot/P-278]

<6 P's of Porphyria>

Pain in abdomen – most common symptom
Peripheral neuropathy
Psychologial abnormalities
Pink urine

Precipitated by drugs (eg Barbiturates, alcohol, oral contraceptives, sulpha drugs)
Photosensitivity is absent

<Reverse the **'AIP'** you get **'PIA'** which means '**P**hotosensitivity **I**s **A**bsent'>

☑ Patients are not photosensitive in **A**cute **I**ntermittent **P**orphyria.

☑ Patients are photosensitive in all other porphyrias.

29. Benzene Ring: Order of Substituents

< Benzene likes to **ROMP**>

From R group moving around the ring:

R group
Ortho
Meta
Para

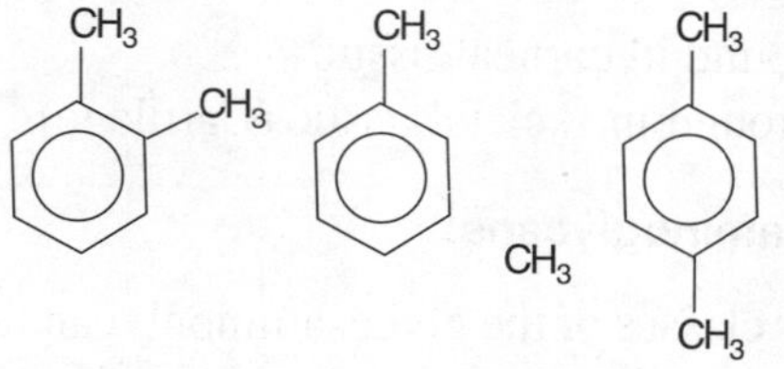

Ortho Meta Para

30. Co-enzyme A: [Harper 25th-621]

<Cozy Pants>

Co-enzyme A is activated **Pant**othenic acid.

Pantothenic acids:

1. Pantothenic acid is formed by combination of Pantoic acid and B-alanine.
2. Active Pantothenic acid is Co-enzyme A (Co-A) and the Acyl carrier protein (ACP)
3. Pantothenic acid deficiency is rare, but occurs in prisoners of war, and, causes *Burning foot syndrome* and is associated with reduced capacity for acetylation.

31. Panthothenic Acid is Needed in:

<FAT Cholesterol>
Fatty acid synthesis (as ACP)
Acetylation reaction (as CoA)
TCA cycle (As CoA)
Cholesterol synthesis.

32. Keratan Sulphate [Lippincot P-149]

<**K**eratan sulphate I is found in the **K**ornea of eye >

Like other glycosaminoglycans keratan sulfate is a linear polymer that consists of a repeating disaccharide unit. Keratan sulfate occurs as a proteoglycan (PG) in which KS chains are attached to cell-surface or extracellular matrix proteins, termed core proteins. KS core proteins include Lumican, Keratocan, Mimecan, Fibromodulin, PRELP, Osteoadherin and Aggrecan.

☑ KS I is found in corneal tissue
☑ KS II is found in skeletal tissue (Cartilage)

33. Glycosaminoglycans:

The 6 major classes of the glycosaminoglycan family vary in the type of hexosamine, hexose or hexuronic acid unit they contain (e.g. glucuronic acid, iduronic acid, galactose, galactosamine, glucosamine).
See table 2.1

Table 2.1

Name	*Hexuronic acid / Hexose*	*Hexosamine*	*Linkage geometry between predominant monomeric units*	*Unique features*
Chondroitin sulfate	GlcUA or GlcUA(2S)	GalNAc or GalNAc(4S) or GalNAc(6S) or GalNAc(4S,6S)	-4GlcUAβ1 -3GalNAcβ1-	Most prevalent GAG
Dermatan sulfate	GlcUA or IdoUA or IdoUA(2S)	GalNAc or GalNAc(4S) or GalNAc(6S) or GalNAc(4S,6S)	-4IdoUAβ1 -3GalNAcβ1-	Distinguished from chondroitin sulfate by the presence of iduronic acid, although some hexuronic acid monosaccharides may be glucuronic acid.
Keratan sulfate	Gal or Gal(6S)	GlcNAc or GlcNAc(6S)	-3Gal(6S)β1 -4GlcNAc(6S)β1-	Keratan sulfate type II may be fucosylated.
Heparin	GlcUA or IdoUA(2S)	GlcNAc or GlcNS or GlcNAc(6S) or GlcNS(6S)	-4IdoUA(2S)α1- 4GlcNS(6S)α1-	Highest negative charge density of any known biological molecule Intracellular component of mast cells

Contd.

Contd.

Heparan sulfate	GlcUA or IdoUA or IdoUA(2S)	GlcNAc or GlcNS or GlcNAc(6S) or GlcNS(6S)	-4GlcUAβ1-4GlcNAcα1-	Highly similar in structure to heparin, however heparan sulfates disaccharide units are organised into distinct sulfated and non-sulfated domains.
Hyaluronan	GlcUA	GlcNAc	-4GlcUAβ1 -3GlcNAcβ1-	The only GAG that is exclusively non-sulfated

Abbreviations:

- GlcUA = β-D-glucuronic acid
- GlcUA(2S) = 2-O-sulfo-β-D-glucuronic acid
- IdoUA = α-L-iduronic acid
- IdoUA(2S) = 2-O-sulfo-α-L-iduronic acid
- Gal = β-D-galactose
- Gal(6S) = 6-O-sulfo-β-D-galactose
- GalNAc = β-D-N-acetylgalactosamine
- GalNAc(4S) = β-D-N-acetylgalactosamine-4-O-sulfate
- GalNAc(6S) = β-D-N-acetylgalactosamine-6-O-sulfate
- GalNAc(4S,6S) = β-D-N-acetylgalactosamine-4-O, 6-O-sulfate
- GlcNAc = α-D-N-acetylglucosamine
- GlcNS = α-D-N-sulfoglucosamine
- GlcNS(6S) = α-D-N-sulfoglucosamine-6-O-sulfate

MULTIPLE CHOICE QUESTIONS

1. **Most common metabolite of progesterone excreted in urine:**
   A. Pregnanelone B. Pregnanetriol
   C. 17-hydroxy pregnanolone D. Pregnanediol
2. **Which of the following is known as suicidal enzyme?**
   A. Lipoxygenase
   B. Cyclooxygenase
   C. Thromboxane synthatase
   D. 5' nucleotidase
3. **All of the following are the reasons responsible for ketosis in a patient of Von-Gierkes disease except:**
   A. They have hypoglycemia
   B. Have low blood sugar levels
   C. Oxaloacetate is required for gluconeogenesis
   D. Low fat mobilization
4. **Exact location of a genetic loci is identified by:**
   A. Fluorescent in-situ hybridization
   B. Polymerase chain reaction
   C. Chromosome painting
   D. Comparative genomic hybridization
5. **True about RIBOZYME:**
   A. Peptidyl transferase activity
   B. Cut DNA at specific site
   C. Participate in DNA synthesis
   D. GTPase activity
6. **Which enzyme's activity is increased in low insulin/glucagon level?**
   A. Hexokinase
   B. Glucokinase
   C. Glucose-6-phosphatase
   D. Pyruvate kinase
7. **Which of the following is false about NADPH?**
   A. Produces ATP in RBCs
   B. Glucose-6-phosphate dehydrogenase causes decreased synthesis of NADPH

C. Required for reductive biosynthesis
D. Stabilizes the membrane of RBCs

8. **Which of the following enzyme is not a component of fatty acid synthase complex?**
   A. Acetyl Co-A carboxylase
   B. Ketoacyl synthase
   C. Enoyl reductase
   D. Acetoacetyl transferase
9. **Ketone bodies can be utilized by all of the following except:**
   A. Skeletal muscle B. Red blood cells
   C. Brain D. Heart
10. **Which of the following is known as suicidal enzyme?**
    A. Lipoxygenase B. Cyclooxygenase
    C. Thromboxane synthatase D. 5' nucleotidase
11. **A child presented with hepatosplenomegaly and pancytopenia. On bone marrow biopsy, large cells with crumpled tissue paper appearance is seen. This is due to deposition of:**
    A. Spingolipids B. Gulcocerebroside
    C. Ceramidate D. Sulphatide
12. **In steps of glycolysis, irreversible enzymes are:**
    A. Hexokinase, pyruvate kinase and phosphofructokinase
    B. Glucokinase, Pyruvate kinase, Glyceraldehyde phosphate dehydrogenase
    C. Pyruvate kinase, Pyruvate caeboxykinase, Hexokinase
    D. Pyruvate kinase, Phosphofructokinase, Fructose 1,6-bisphosphate
13. **All of the following are the reasons responsible for ketosis in a patient of Von-Gierkes disease except:**
    A. They have hypoglycemia
    B. Have low blood sugar levels
    C. Oxaloacetate is required for gluconeogenesis
    D. Low fat mobilization
14. **Exact location of a genetic loci is identified by:**

A. Fluorescent in-situ hybridization
B. Polymerase chain reaction
C. Chromosome painting
D. Comparative genomic hybridization

15. Which of the following enzyme is not involved in oxidation-reduction reaction?
A. Oxygenase B. Hydrolases
C. Hydroperoxidase D. Dehydrogenase

16. Long chain fatty acid transported into inner mitochondria membrane by:
A. Acyl carrier protein
B. Acyl carnitine
C. Simple diffusion
D. Energy mediated

17. The primary role of chaperones is to help in:
A. Protein synthesis
B. Protein degradation
C. Protein denaturation
D. Protein folding

18. β-oxidation of odd-chain fatty acids produces:
A. Succinyl CoA
B. Propionyl CoA
C. Acetyl CoA
D. Malonyl CoA

19. The buffering capacity of a buffer is maximum at pH equal to:
A. 0.5 pKa **B.** pKa
C. pKa + 1 **D.** 2 pKa

20. Which of the following is not a post-transcriptional modification of RNA?
A. Splicing
B. 5' capping
C. 3' polyadenylation
D. Glycosylation

21. Accumulation of sphingomyelin in phagocytic cells is a feature of:
A. Gaucher disease
B. Niemann-Pick disease
C. Tay-Sachs disease
D. Down syndrome

22. **Which one of the following pairs of lipids and related compounds exhibit opposite biologic activities?**
    A. 5-HPETE and leukotriene D4
    B. Cholic acid and lithocolic acid
    C. Thromboxane A2 and prostacyclin (PGI2)
    D. Acetone and beta—hydroxybutyrate
23. **Enzyme deficient in Type-1 Hyperlipidemia is:**
    A. HMG CoA reductase
    B. Lipoprotein lipase
    C. Cholesterol acyl transferase
    D. Peroxidase
24. **In porphyra cutanea tarda the type of porphyrin excreted in urine is:**
    A. Coproporphyrin-I
    B. Uroporphyrin-I
    C. Uroporphyrin-II
    D. Type I and III uroporphyrins
25. **In competitive inhibition the relation of Km and Vmax is one of the following:**
    A. Km and Vmax are the same
    B. Km increases and Vmax is the same
    C. Km decreases and Vmax increases
    D. Km and Vmax decreases
26. **Amino acid used in the synthesis of purines:**
    A. Glycine
    B. Ornithine
    C. Alanine
    D. Threonine
27. **Km of an enzyme is:**
    A. Dissociation constant
    B. The normal physiological substrate concentration
    C. The substrate concentration at half maximum velocity
    D. Numerically identical for all isozymes that catalyze a given reaction
28. **What is the connecting link between urea cycle and TCA cycle?**
    A. Fumarate
    B. Succinate

C. Oxaloacetate
D. Arginino succinate

29. **Protein acts as buffer due to which property?**
A. Colloid
B. Basic
C. Acidic
D. Amphipathic (amphoteric in nature)

30. **Which of the following amino acids is associated with increased risk of Myocardial Infarction?**
A. Methionine
B. Homocysteine
C. Ornithine
D. Valine

31. **When the following amino acids are separated by running them on agarose gel, at pH 7, which one of them will migrate slowest to the anodic end?**
A. Glycine
B. Valine
C. Aspartic acid
D. Lysine

32. **On complete hydrolysis of DNA we will get all the following *except*:**
A. Deoxy pentose sugar
B. Phosphoric acid
C. Adenosine
D. Purine bases

33. **What is the technique by which DNA can be amplified?**
A. Southern blot
B. Polymerase chain reaction
C. Hybridization
D. Western blot

34. **Km increases but Vmax same—enzyme is:**
A. Competitive
B. Non-competitive
C. Irreversible
D. Uncompetitive

35. **Familial hypercholesterolemia is:**
A. Deficient LDL receptors
B. Deficient HDL receptors

C. HMG CoA reductase deficiency
D. Deficient VLDL receptors

36. **Which one is nonsense codon?**
A. UUA
B. UAG
C. UGA
D. UAU

37. **Visualisation of specific RNA fragment using RNA probe is:**
A. Southern blotting
B. Western blotting
C. Eastern blotting
D. Northern blotting

38. **Which is true regarding nitric oxide in human beings?**
A. Produced from nitrous oxide
B. Produced only in macrophage
C. Potent vasoconstrictor
D. Potent vasodilator effect

39. **Not produced in Adrenaline synthesis pathway:**
A. DOPA
B. Dopamine
C. Nor adrenaline
D. Tyramine

40. **Which one of the following is the correct sequential order in which the given enzymes of Kreb's cycle are formed after a molecule of acetyl CoA enters the cycle?**
A. Citrate, Oxaloacetate, Ketoglutarate
B. Ketoglutarate, Oxalocetate, Citrate
C. Citrate, Ketoglutatrate, Oxalocetate
D. Oxaloacetate, Ketoglutarate, Citrate

41. **Indole ring is present in:**
A. Tryptophan
B. Valine
C. Methionine
D. Histidine

42. **Gilberts syndrome disease all are true, *except*:**
A. Conjugated hyperbilirubinemia

B. Fasting hypoglycaemia
C. Normal liver history
D. Liver enzymes normal

43. Fidelity enzyme in protein synthesis:
A. DNA polymerase
B. RNA polymerase
C. Amino-acyl tRNA synthase
D. Amino acyl reductase

44. Pyruvate dehydrogenase contains all *except*:
A. Biotin
B. NAD
C. FAD
D. CoA

45. Thyroxine and catecholamine are derived from:
A. Tyrosine
B. Typtophan
C. Alanine
D. Leucine

46. Fluroacetate inhibits:
A. Citrate synthetase
B. Aconitase
C. Succinic dehydrogenase
D. Alphaketoglutarate dehydrogenase

47. Heart uses one of following as energy source during starvation:
A. Glucose
B. Acetoacetate
C. Fats
D. Proteins

48. Muscle is not involved in which type of glycogen storage disease?
A. Type I
B. Type II
C. Type III
D. Type IV

49. Oxidation of fatty acids occur in:
A. Cytoplasm
B. Ribosomes
C. Centrioles
D. Mitochondria

50. **Thermostability of DNA is provided by:**
   A. G-C bonds
   B. A-T paining
   C. N-glycosolic bond
   D. Antiparallel arrangement
51. **Vitamin necessary for CoA synthesis:**
   A. Pantothenic acid
   B. Vit C
   C. B_4
   D. Biotin
52. **Dietary fibre is rich in:**
   A. Starch
   B. Pectin
   C. Collagen
   D. Proteoglycan
53. **The following is neuro transmitter:**
   A. Serine
   B. Glutathione
   C. Glutamine
   D. Glutamate
54. **Non-essential amino acid is:**
   A. Tyrosine
   B. Phenyalanine
   C. Lysine
   D. Threonine
55. **Part of M-RNA removed during protein synthesis:**
   A. Intron
   B. Codon
   C. Exon
   D. Cistron
56. **Metabolite of epinephrine is:**
   A. Metanephrine
   B. Nor metanephrine
   C. Hydroxy mandelic acid
   D. 3 methoxy-2 hydroxy glycol
57. **Examples of monounsaturated fatty acids are:**
   A. Oleic acid
   B. Arachidonic acid
   C. Linolenic acid
   D. Palmitic acid

58. **Acidic amino acids are:**
A. Asparagine
B. Arginine
C. Glutamine
D. Lysine
E. None

59. **Aromatic amino acids are:**
A. Tryptophan
B. Tyrosine
C. Lysine
D. Arginine
E. Phenylalanine

60. **All these reactions take place inside the mitochondria *except*:**
A. EM pathway
B. Krebs cycle
C. Urea cycle
D. Electron transfer
E. Fatty acid cycle of oxidation

61. **Specific poison for succinate dehydrogenase is:**
A. Cyanide
B. Malonate
C. Arsenite
D. Fluoride
E. Malate

62. **What is the average number of high energy bonds required for the synthesis of 1 peptide bond?**
A. 1
B. 2
C. 3
D. 4
E. 5

63. **Which is the by product of urea cycle?**
A. Aspartate
B. Succinate
C. Ornithine
D. Fumarate

64. **Succinyl CoA is produced by all *except*:**
A. Isoleucine
B. Methionine

C. Valine
D. Phenylalanine

65. Amino acids excreted in urine in Maple Syrup urine disease are all *except*:
A. Isoleucine B. Valine
C. Lysine D. Leucine

66. High energy compound which does not have phosphate:
A. SAM
B. AMP
C. c-AMP
D. GTP

67. Amino acids excreted in urine in cystinuria *except*:
A. Lysine
B. Arginine
C. Ornithine
D. Cystine
E. None

68. Number of ATP used in glycolysis:
A. 2 B. 1
C. 8 D. 10
E. None

69. All are produced from tyrosine *except*:
A. DOPA
B. Serotonin
C. Maleylacetoacetate
D. Melanin

ANSWERS

1. **D.** Pregnanediol
2. **B.** Cyclooxygenase
3. **D.** Low fat mobilization
4. **A.** Fluorescent in-situ hybridization
5. **A.** Peptidyl transferase activity
6. **C.** Glucose-6-phosphatase
7. **A.** Produces ATP in RBCs
8. **A.** Acetyl Co-A carboxylase
9. **B.** Red blood cells
10. **B.** Cyclooxygenase
11. **B.** Gulcocerebroside
12. **A.** Hexokinase, pyruvate kinase and phosphofructokinase
13. **D.** Low fat mobilization
14. **A.** Fluorescent in-situ hybridization
15. **B.** Hydrolases
16. **B.** Acyl carnitine
17. **D.** Protein folding
18. **B.** Propionyl CoA
19. **B.** pKa
20. **D.** Glycosylation
21. **B.** Niemann-Pick Disease
22. **C.** Thromboxane A_2 and prostacyclin (PGI_2)
23. **B.** Lipoprotein lipase
24. **D.** Type I and III uroporphyrins
25. **B.** Km increases and V_{max} is the same
26. **A.** Glycine
27. **C.** The substrate concentration at half maximum velocity
28. **A.** Fumarate
29. **D.** Amphipathic (amphoteric in nature)
30. **B.** Homocysteine
31. **D.** Lysine
32. **C.** Adenosine
33. **B.** Polymerase chain reaction
34. **A.** Competitive
35. **A.** Deficient LDL receptors
36. **B.** UAG
    C. UGA

37. **D.** Northern blotting
38. **D.** Potent vasodilator effect
39. **D.** Tyramine
40. **C.** Citrate, Ketoglutarate, Oxalocetate
41. **A.** Tryptophan
42. **A.** Conjugated hyperbilirubinemia
43. **C.** Amino-acyl tRNA synthase
44. **A.** Biotin
45. **A.** Tyrosine
46. **B.** Aconitase
47. **B.** Acetoacetate
48. **A.** Type I
49. **D.** Mitochondria
50. **A.** G-C bonds
51. **A.** Pantothenic acid
52. **B.** Pectin
53. **D.** Glutamate
54. **A.** Tyrosine
55. **A.** Intron
56. **A.** Metanephrine
57. **A.** Oleic acid
58. **E.** None
59. **A.** Tryptophan
    B. Tyrosine
    E. Phenylalanine
60. **A.** EM pathway
61. **B.** Malonate
62. **D.** 4
63. **D.** Funmarate
64. **D.** Phenylalanine
65. **C.** Lysine
66. **A.** SAM
67. **E.** None
68. **A.** 2
69. **B.** Serotonin

3 *Physiology*

I. CIRCULATION

1. Erythropoiesis: Stages [S.K. Chaudhuri 2nd—28]

"**P**rofitable **B**usinesses **P**ollute **O**ur **R**ural **E**nvironment"
Pronormoblast (Proerythroblast) (E_1)
Basophilic normoblast (E_2)
Polychromatophilic normoblast (E_4)
Orthochromatic normoblast (E_5)
Reticulocyte (E_6)
Erythrocytes (E_7).
<**P**rivate **B**usinessmen **P**ollute **O**ur **R**ural **E**nvironment>

2. White Blood Cells: Types and Percentage

"**N**aughty **L**ittle **M**onkeys **E**ating **B**ananas"
Neutrophils (65%)
Lymphocytes (35%)
Monocytes (6%)
Eosinophils (3%)
Basophils (1%).

3. Coagulation Common Pathway: Factors in Order [G-545]

<10 + 5 - 2 = 13>
Coagulation common pathway:
Factor **X** → Factor **V** → Factor **II** → Factor **XIII** **(Fig. 3.1).**

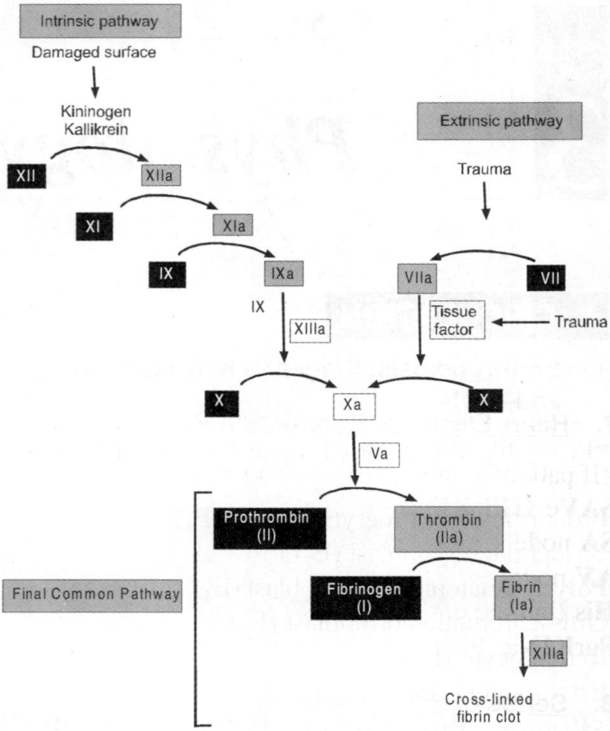

Fig. 3.1: Clotting cascade

4. PT vs. PTT [R-649]

Long name—Long path [PTT for intrinsic path]
Short name—Short path [PT for extrinsic path].

5. PGI_2 vs. TxA_2 Coagulation Function [R-69]

Tx**A**$_2$: **A**ggregates platelets.
PG**I**$_2$: **I**nhibits platelet aggregation.

6. Einthoven's Triangle: Organization [G-555]

<The keyword is **L**>

☑ Corners are at RA (right arm), LA (left arm), LL (left leg).

☑ Number of L's at a corner tell how many + signs are at that corner [e.g. LL is ++].

☑ Sum of number of L's of any 2 corners tells the name of the lead [e.g. LL-LA is lead III].

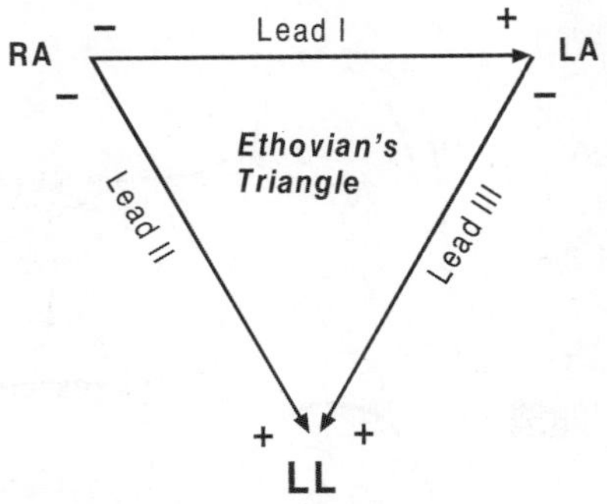

Fig. 3.2

7. Heart Electrical Conduction Pathway

<If patient's family is having heart attacks, you must **SAVe HIS KIN**!>

SA node
AV node
His (bundle of)
Pur**KIN**je fibers.

8. Series of Events in Heart

p	a	q	1	c	2	v	3	p	a
			r	x			y		4

First Write p a................p a

☑ Then insert q c v Corners are at RA (right arm), LA (left arm), LL (left leg).

Then write 123

Then the corresponding r x y 4

☑ a,c,v,x,y are jugular venous pulsations

☑ p,q,r are ECG waves

☑ 1,2,3,4 are heart sounds.

See Fig. 3.3 on next page.

9. Wenckebach's Phenomenon [Ganong 22nd Ed/P-555]

<Wen-Ke-Back>

When the P-R interval **Keeps** on prolonging, the heart drops **Back** a beat and the cardiac cycle goes **Back** to normal length.

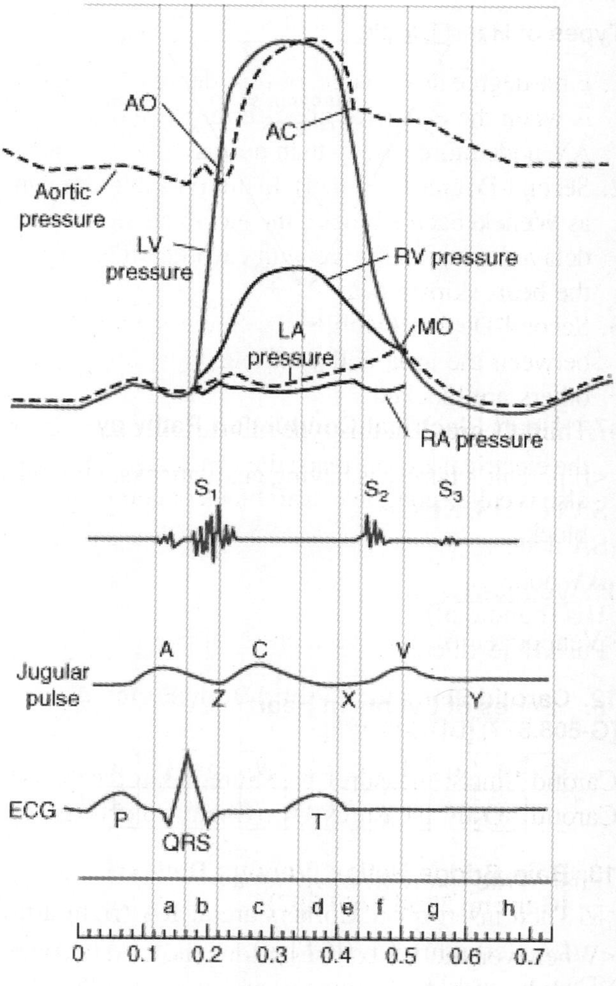

Fig. 3.3

It is seen in second degree heart block (Mobitz Type I).

10. Strokes Adam Syndrome [Ganong 22nd Ed/P-555]

<Poor **Adam** faints, whenever he has a heart **Stroke**>

Strokes Adam syndrome is characterized by repeated fainting attacks associated with complete (third degree) heart block.

Types of Heart Block:

1. First-degree heart block, or first-degree AV block, is when the electrical impulse moves through the AV node more slowly than normal.
2. Second-Degree (Mobitz I): In this type (also known as Wenckebach's block), the electrical signals are delayed more and more with each heartbeat, until the heart skips a beat.
3. Second-Degree (Mobitz II): Some signals move between the atria and ventricles normally, while others are blocked.
4. Third Degree : In this type of heart block, none of the electrical signals reach the ventricles. This type also is called complete heart block or complete AV block.

11. Venous Return:

<Venous return: **I**ncreases on **I**nspiration>

12. Carotid Sinus vs. Carotid Body Function [G-608,677] [BDC-III-102]

Carotid **S**inu**S**: measures pre**SS**ure. (Baroreceptors)
Carotid b**O$_2$**dy measures **O$_2$**. (Chemoreceptors)

13. Bain Bridge Reflex (Venous Reflex) [Ganong 22nd Ed/P-607]

<Whenever the water rises under the bridge, poor Bain's heart starts beating fast and he makes the great escape>

Bain bridge reflex is characterized by reflex increase in the rate on venous engorgement of the right atrium and right great veins. Vagus escape is mediated by Bainbridge reflex.

Cardiovascular reflexes

The cardiovascular system is centrally regulated by automatic reflexes. These work with local mechanisms to minimize fluctuations in the mean arterial blood pressure (MABP) and to maintain adequate perfusion of each organ. Intrinsic reflexes

Contd.

Contd.

respond to stimuli originating from within the cardiovascular system. These include the baroreceptor, cardiopulmonary and chemoreceptor reflexes, and their properties are summarized in table below. The extrinsic reflexes mediate the cardiovascular response to stimuli originating from for example pain and temperature changes.

Reflexes involve three components:

1. Afferent nerves sense a change in the state of the system, and communicate this to the brain
2. The brain process this information and implements an appropriate response
3. Which results in altering the activity of efferent nerves controlling cardiac and pulmonary function, thereby causing homeostatic response that reverse the change in state

Intrinsic Cardiovascular Reflexes

Receptors Reflex Location	*Stimulated By*	*Response Activated*
Arterial baroreceptors; carotid sinus and aortic arch	Change in arterial blood pressure, affects degree of stretch of arterial wall	If pressure decreases: vagal and sympathetic tachycardia; sympathetic vasoconstriction; renin release. If pressure increases opposite effects.
Cardiopulmonary receptors: • Atrial mechanoreceptors / Bainbridge reflex • Atrial nonmyelinated vagal efferents • Ventricular and coronary nonmyelinated vagal efferents	Change in blood volume and pressure in central thoracic compartment; affects degree of stretch of atria, ventricles, coronary arteries	Net effect: Decrease in pressure and volume: Sympathetic and/or vagal tachycardia; vasoconstriction; venoconstriction; reduced production of urine Opposite with volume and pressure increase
☑ Venticular chemoreceptors / Bezold-Jarisch effect	Cardiac ischeamia, drugs	Bradycardia; vasodilation

Contd.

Contd.

☑ J-receptors / Lung	Marked lung inflation, pulmonary congestion	Tachycardia; vasodilation
Arterial chemoreceptors: carotid sinus and aortic arch	Severe hypotension, hypoxia, asphyxia causing decreased pO_2, increased pCO_2 and H+ in blood	Sympathetic vasoconstriction; indirect tachycardia; stimulation of respiration
CNS ischeamic response/ Cushing reflex	Brainstem ischeamia	Sympathetic peripheral vasoconstriction
Extrinsic Reflexes Stimuli that are external to the cardiovascular system also exert effects on the heart and vasculature via extrinsic reflexes. Moderate pain causes tachycardia and increases in MABP. Severe pain has the opposite effect. Cold causes cutaneous and coronary vasoconstriction, possibly precipitating angina in susceptible individuals.		

14. <u>Atrial Fibrillation and Flutter</u> [Ganong 22nd-557]

<Fibrillation is a longer word than flutter>
So the heart rate must be more in fibrillation (>300) than flutter (200-350).

15. <u>Oculocardiac Reflex</u> [Ganong 22nd-557]

<Where do you **see** things which are loved by the **heart** ? … Of course in Las **Vegas**>

☑ On pressing the eyeball tachycardia can often be converted to normal sinus rhythm. This is called oculocardiac reflex and it is mediated by vagus nerve.

16. <u>Second Heart Sound</u> [SKC- 217]

<**S**econd heart sound is **S**hort and **S**harp>
<PALE>
Pulmonary valve closes – **L**ate.
Aortic valve closes – **E**arly.
<AttaPattu (A2P2)>
A_2 occurs slightly before P_2.

17. Hb-oxygen Dissociation Curve Shifts: Effect, Location [G-670]

Left shift: causes **L**oading of O_2 in **L**ungs from Hb. (↑O_2 affinity)
Right shift: causes **R**elease of O_2 from **R**BC (Hb). (?O_2 affinity)

18. Hemoglobin Binding Curve: Causes of Shift to Right [Ganong 20th Ed/P-670]

<**CADET**, face right **!**>
CO_2
Acid/**A**ltitude
2,3-**D**PG
Exercise
Temperature
When any of the above factors is increased there is right shift in the hemoglobin binding curve.
See Fig. 3.4

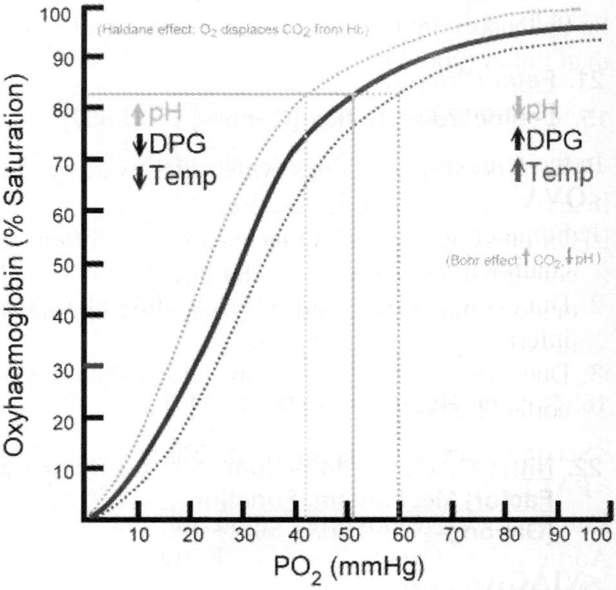

Fig. 3.4

19. Alkalosis vs. Acidosis: Directions of pH and HCO_3

<ROME>

Respiratory= **O**pposite:		
Acidosis	pH is ↓	PCO_2 is ↑
Alkalosis	pH is ↑	PCO_2 is ↓
Metabolic= **E**qual:		
Acidosis	pH is ↓	HCO_3 is ↓
Alkalosis	pH is ↑	HCO_3 is ↑ ().

20. Blood Flow and Oxygen Consumption of Important Organs [Ganong 22nd Ed/P-621]

☑ Liver is the largest organ so it enjoys the maximum blood flow (1500 mL/min) and maximum oxygen consumption (51 mL/min) on the whole.

☑ Heart is near the lungs so it steals a lot of oxygen and is also a spendthrift: Max AV oxygen difference (114 mL/L) and max O_2 consumption per 100g of tissue (9.7 mL/100g/min).

☑ The small Kidney is near the liver so it gets a lot of blood: Maximum blood flow per 100 g of tissue (420 mL/100g/min).

21. Fetal Circulation [Ganong 22nd– 628, SKC–367]

In the fetus there are 3 bypass channels:
<OVA>

1. Foramen **o**vale: Connecting right→left atrium (2 chambers).
2. Ductus **v**enosus: Connecting umbilical vein→ inferior vena cava (2 veins).
3. Ductus **a**rteriosus: Connecting pulmonary artery→ aorta (2 arteries).

22. Nitric Oxide (Endothelium Derived Relaxing Factor) Mechanism, Function [Ganong—22nd Ed/P_598]

<VIAGRA>
Vasodilation

Inhibited by hemoglobin
Activated by agents that cause increase in intracellular Ca^{++}
c**G**MP increased in smooth muscles
Relax smooth muscle
Arginine (Synthesized from arginine).

☑ Nitric oxide is the vasodilator transmitter substance at the parasympathetic penile nerve endings which cause erection, hence "VIAGRA".

< Nitric oxide synthase is found in **MEN** >
Macrophages
Endothelial cells
Nervous system

Also remember:

Nitric oxide synthase (NOS)

Type	*Found in*
1	**N**ervous system
2	**M**acrophages
3	**E**ndothelial cells

Venous return: **I**ncreases on **I**nspiration

II. ENDOCRINE, METABOLISM AND REPRODUCTION

1. Adrenal Cortex Layers and Products [G-360]

Layers: **<GFR>**
Glomerulosa (outermost)
Fasiculata
Reticulata
Respective products:
<It gets sweeter as you go deeper>
Mineralcorticoids
Glucocorticoids
Sex hormones.
Alternatively:
<Go Find Rex, Make Good Sex>

2. Diabetes Insipidus: Diagnosing Subtypes [H-2099]

After a desmopression injection:
Concentrated urine = **C**ranial.
No effect = **N**ephrogenic.

3. Progesterone: Actions [G-447]

<PROGEST>
Produce cervical mucous
Relax uterine smooth muscle
Oxycotin sensitivity down
Gonadotropin [FSH, LH] secretions down
Endometrial spiral arteries and secretions up
Sustain pregnancy
Temperature up/**T**it (breast) development.

4. Hormonal Picture at the Time of Ovulation: [Shaws 12th Ed/P--37]

<HELP me in this **surge>**
High **E**strogen **L**ow **P**rogestrone occurs during **LH Surge** which causes **ovulation**.

5. Prolactin and Oxytocin: Functions [G-250,426]

PROlactin stimulates the mammary glands to **PRO**duce milk.
Oxytocin stimulates the mammary glands to **O**oze (release) milk. (Milk ejection reflex)

6. Hormones Secreted by Sartoli Cells [SKC - 343]

<AIM>
Androgen binding protein
Inhibin
Mullerian inhibiting substance
Other functions of sartoli cells:
< 4P's >
Provide nutrition to developing sperm cells
Phagocytoze injured or dead sperm cells
Prevents substances from entering the lumen of seminiferous tubules (Blood testis barrier)
Produce some estrogen from testosterone.

7. Sartoli vs. Leydig Cells: [SKC/P-243]

- **Sartoli** cells:
  <**Sort** out the **Sex** confusion>
  Secretes Mullerian inhibiting substance and
  It is present only in **Sirs** (males).
- **Leydig cells** :
  <You need real **Testosterone** to ***lay*** and ***dig*** her>
  Leydig cells secrete testosterone.

8. Hormones of Pituitary Gland [Ganong 20th Ed/P-383]

<GOAT FLAP>
1. **G**rowth hormone
2. **O**xytocin – *Posterior pituitary*
3. **A**denocorticotropin (ACTH)
4. **T**hyroid stimulating hormone
5. **F**ollicle stimulating hormone
6. **L**uteinizing hormone

7. **A**nti-diuretic hormone (Vasopressin) – *Posterior pituitary*
8. **P**rolactin

See Fig. 3.5

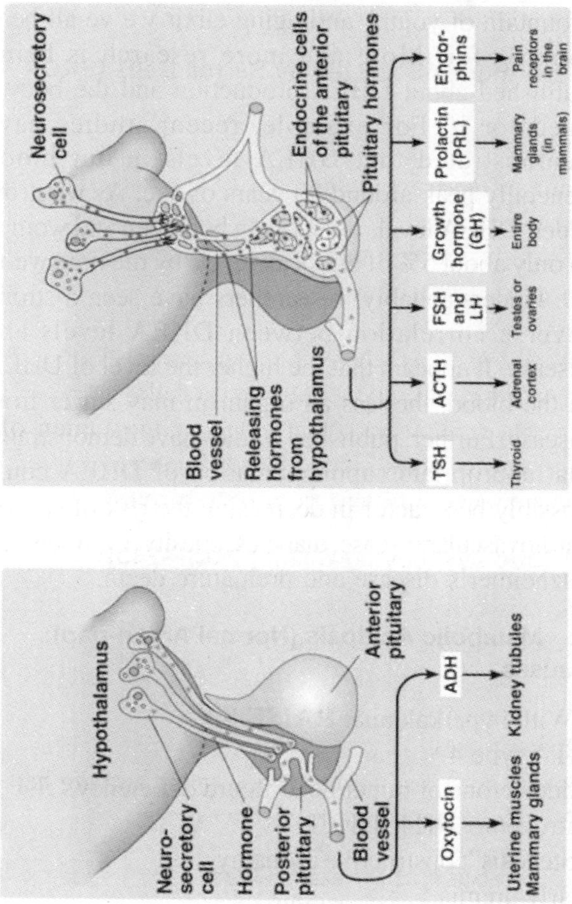

Fig. 3.5

8. What is DHEA?

DHEA (or dehydroepiandrosterone) is commonly called the "mother" hormone, since from it a number of other hormones may be manufactured upon demand, such as estrogen, testosterone, progesterone and corticosterone to name just a few. Because of DHEA's biochemical flexibility, it has become the subject of much recent study, especially for its almost unbelievable but wonderful potential to actually slow the aging process. Some are even calling it the "fountain of youth" anti-aging elixir we've all been looking for. More and more research is being published about DHEA production and the body's need for it. For example, recent studies have demonstrated that DHEA levels in our blood generally peak around 20 years of age. As we grow older, DHEA levels decrease in both men and women to only about 5% of our peak levels by the time we're 80. Understandably, researchers have seen a strong inverse correlation between DHEA levels and disease. It appears that the higher the level of DHEA in the blood, the less an organism may suffer from disease. Further, published studies have demonstrated that appropriate supplementation of DHEA could possibly be a factor in decreasing the risk of cancer, cardiovascular disease, diabetes, obesity, even senility, Alzheimer's disease and premature death.

9. Metabolic Acidosis (Normal Anion-gap): Causes

<With hyperkalemia: **RAISE** K+ >
RTA type 4
Aldosterone or mineralocorticord deficiency
Iatrogenic: NH4Cl, HCl
"**S**tenosis": obstructive uropathy
Early uremia

<With hypokalemia: **ReDUCE** K+ >
Renal TA type 1 and 2
Diarrhoea
Urine diversion into gut
Carbonate anhydrase inhibitor
Ex-hyperventilation

10. Galactosaemia: Enzyme Deficiency

<**GALIPUT**: **Gal**actose **1** **P**hosphate **U**ridyl **T**ransferase>

☑ There is an assay called the **Galiput** test for this.

10. Carbon Monoxide: Electron Transport Chain Target

<**"CO blocks CO"**>

Carbon monoxide (CO) blocks Cytochrome Oxidase (CO)

III. NERVES AND MUSCLES

1. Nervous System: Divisions

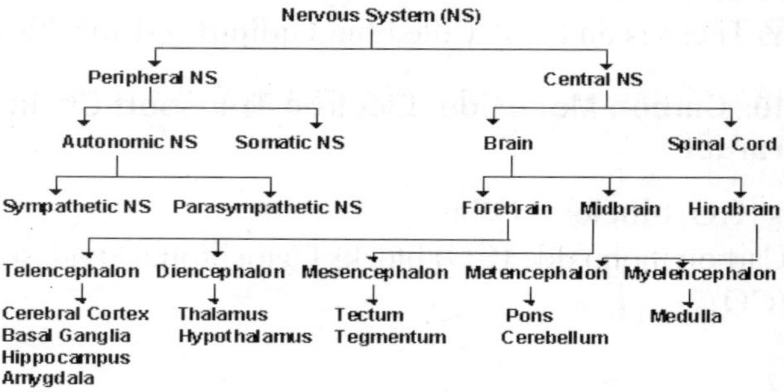

2. Temperature Control: Cerebral Regions [G-257]

"**H**igh **P**ower **A**ir **C**onditioner":
Heating = **P**osterior hypothalamus (causes shivering)
Anterior hypothalamus = **C**ooling (causes cutaneous vasodilatation and sweating)

3. Thirst/Water Balance Control Centre: Location in Hypothalamus

"You look up (supra...optic) at the clouds, to check if it's going to rain (water)>

Therefore, water balance is in **supraoptic** nucleus.

4. Hypothalamus: Feeding vs. Satiety Center

"Stim the lat, get fat":
Stimulating **lat**eral hypothalamus increases hunger: Person becomes fat.
Its destruction causes severe fatal anorexia.

<Stim the ven, get thin>
Stimulating **ven**tromedial hypothalamus increases satiety: Person becomes thin.
Its destruction causes hyperphagia.

5. Urination: Autonomic Control [G-730]

"When you urinate, it's **PIS**s":
Parasympathetic **I**nhibits **S**ympathetic.

6. Penis Autonomic Innervation Actions [BDC-II –307]

"Point and Shoot"
Parasympathetic **P**oints the **P**enis, **S**ympathetic **S**hoots out the **S**emen (Erection and Ejaculation).

Parasympathetic causes **P**otty and **P**ee (defecation and urination).

☑ *Innervation of penis:*
Parasympathetic – S_2,S_3,S_4
Sympathetic - T_{11} to L_2

7. Taste buds: Vallate vs. Fungiform Distribution [Ganong 20th Ed/P-184]

Cross sectional shape of the top of the bud tells their distribution.

Vallate papillae: Have a shallow **'V'** at the top, therefore have a **'V'** shaped distribution at the back of the tongue.

Fungiform papillae: Top is **round** so it is towards the **round end** of the tongue.

☑ Note: Vallate is also sometimes called circumvallate.

<**N**ew **T**aste **S**ensation travel through **N**ucleus **T**ractus **S**olitarius>

8. Taste Sensation Distribution [Ganong 20th Ed/P-184]

a. Bitter: Back of tongue
   - When you take a bitter pill you throw it in your mouth as far as possible.

b. Sour: On sides
   - Imagine the juice of a lemon trickling by the sides of your tongue.

c. Salty: Dorsum of tongue (anteriorly)
   - Imagine taking a pinch of salt and sprinkling it on your tongue.

d. Sweet: At the tip
   - **Imagine licking a sweet candy with the tip of your tongue.**

3. Taste Pathway: [Ganong 20th Ed/P-184]

<**A**nyone **C**an **P**ass **G**as !>
Anterior two third is supplied by **C**horda Tympani (branch of Facial nerve)
Posterior one third is supplied by **G**lossopharyngeal nerve

4. Muscle Sarcomere: A vs. I as light or dark [G-67]

There is only one vowel* in >d**a**rk> – '**a**'
and one vowel in >light> – '**i**'
These one vowels match up to their one letter names:
<D**a**rk band is the **A** band>
<L**i**ght band is the **I** band>

☑ Vowels in english alphabets are "a, e, i, o, and u"

5. Muscle Sarcomere: H line vs. Z disc location [G-67]

< **HAZI** >
H- band is part of A-band.
Z-line is present in the I-band.
☑ H-band disappears during muscle contraction.

See Fig. 3.6.

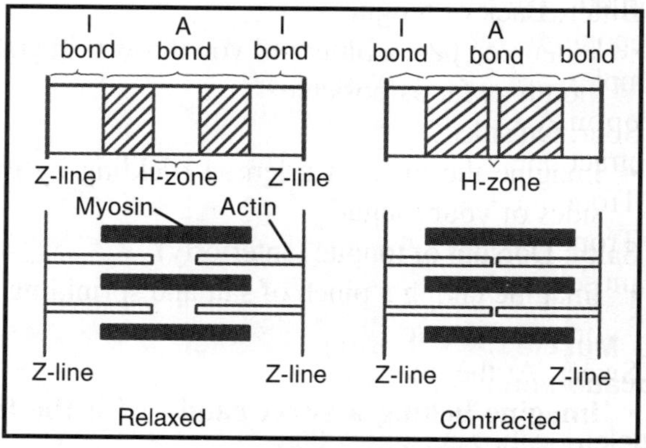

Fig. 3.6

6. Muscle Contraction: [SKC – 507]

<Tropomyosin – **To-Pre-Myosin** >
Tropomyosin is a molecule meant **To Prevent Myosin**. It covers the active site on the thin filament of actin in relaxed state and prevents myosin from attaching to actin.

Events in order during muscle contraction:
1. Action potential on sarcolemma
2. Generation of T-tubule potential
3. Ca^{++} ions release from L-tubules
4. Calcium binding to Troponin C
5. Displacement of Tropomyosin from active site of actin.
6. Attachment of myosin head to active sites of actin F.
7. Power stroke and contraction.

Steps 4 to 7 can be remembered as:
Mnemonic: **<When Tropomyosin goes to C (see) Troponin, Myosin comes and F**** Actin.>**
Also remember: < **L** tubules release ca**L**cium >

7. Troponin Types: [ref. http://herkules.oulu.fi/isbn9514267370/html/x624.html]

<**TIC**>
Troponin **T** – fixes the **T**roponin group to **T**ropomyosin.
Troponin **I** – **I**nhibits ATP-ase activity of acto-myosin complex.
Troponin **C** – binds to **C**alcium and initiates contraction.
☑ Troponin **T** and **I** are **C**ardiac specific <**TIC**>.
☑ Troponin **I** has never been detected in skeletal muscle

8. Muscle Cells: Cardiac vs. Skeletal's Nuclei Location/number [G-79]

Nuclei location mirrors where the muscle is located in human body.

Heart muscle is in the middle of body, so heart muscle cells have nucleus in middle.
Skeletal muscles are at periphery of body, so nuclei are at periphery.
Also know:
You have 1 heart, so there is usually only 1 nucleus per heart muscle cell.
You have many skeletal muscles, so there are many nuclei per long fiber.

9. Lateral Spinothalamic Tract [Ganong 20th- 133]

<PTO>
Pain and Temperature – Opposite
*These are fibers which cross in the spinal cord and hence in lateral injury to the spinal cord, pain and temperature of opposite half of the body is lost below the site of injury.

10. Spinal tracts: Gracilus vs. Cuneatus: Origin from Upper vs. Lower Limbs

Gracilus is the name of a muscle in the legs, so Fasciculus Gracilus is for the lower limbs.
Therefore Fasciculus Cuneatus must be for upper limbs.
See next page for Fig. 3.7

11. Types of Waves in EEG [Ganong 22nd Ed/P-195, Neeraj Ahuja P-141]

<To Increase your mental frequency take ***D-TAB*****>**
*(**D**elta, **T**heta, **A**lpha, **B**eta)*
—Frequency increases from delta to beta.
—Amplitude has inverse relation with frequency, i.e. amplitude decreases as frequency increases.
δ-waves – 0.5 to 3 Hz
θ-waves – 4 to 7 Hz
α-waves – 8 to 12 Hz
β-waves – 18 to 30 Hz

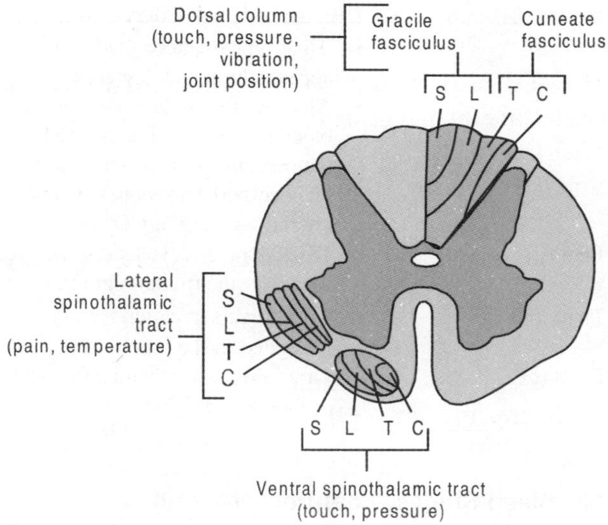

Fig. 3.7: Cross-section of spinal cord, showing location of ascending sensory pathways. Note that each is laminated. S, sacral; L, lumbar; T, thoracic; C, cervical

☑ A German psychiatrist Hans Berger introduced the term EEG.

☑ The electrocorticogram (ECoG) is used to refer to the record obtained with the electrodes on the pial surface of the cortex.

☑ When the attention is focused on something, the alpha wave is replaced by fast, somewhat irregular low voltage activity. This phenomenon is called as alpha block.

☑ During active mental concentration beta like rhythm and sometimes gamma rhythm is seen.

Rhythm	*Remarks*
Alpha (α)	• Seen at rest with eyes closed and mind wandering. • Regular pattern with frequency 8-12/s; Amplitude of 50 mV. • Most marked in parieto-occipital region.

Contd.

Contd.

	• Adult alpha pattern gradually appears during adolescence. • Alpha rhythm is decreased by a low blood glucose level; a low body temperature; a low level of adrenal glucocorticoid hormones; a high arterial pressure of CO_2 .
Beta (β)	• 18 - 30/s, of lower voltage, sometimes seen over the frontal regions.
Theta (θ)	• 4-7/s, occurs in children and is generated in the hippocampus.
Delta (δ)	• Large slow waves with a frequency of less than 4/s.

12. Sleep Stages: Features [NA-140]

<**DE**lta waves during **DE**epest sleep (stages 3 & 4, slow-wave)>

<d**RE**a**M** occur during **REM** sleep>

13. Parasomnias (Sleep Disorders) [NA-148, Ganong 22nd -201]

SLeep terrors (Night terror) and **SL**eepwalking occur during **SL**ow-wave sleep (stage 4).

Nightma**RE** occurs during **REM** sleep and is **REM**embered.

☑ Note – Night terrors are not remembered and occur in NREM sleep

<NREM – WET>

Walking

Eneuresis

Terror / **T**alking / **T**eeth grinding

(All this occur in NREM sleep)

14. CSF Circulation: Function of Choroid vs. Arachnoid Granules

Choroid **C**reates CSF.

Arachnoid granules **A**bsorb CSF.

15. Geniculate Bodies: Medial vs. Lateral System [Ganong-20th -168]

<MALE>
Medial=**A**uditory
Lateral=**E**ye.
Medial geniculate body is for auditory system, lateral geniculate body is for visual system.
Can expand to <**MALES**> to remember **L**ateral=**E**ye=**S**uperior colliculus (thus medial is inferior colliculus by default).

16. Language Disorders: [Ganong 22nd – 274, Fig-16.6]

a. <**Broca**>: your speech machinery is **Broken.** In Broca's aphasia (nonfluent aphasia) speech is slow and hard to come by. Patient is limited to only few words.
b. <**Wer-nick**>: "**were**" and "**nick**" are both words of English language, but together they are nonsensical.
In Wernicke's aphasia, speech itself is normal and patient talks excessively, but says words that don't make sense together. Patient also fails to comprehend the meaning of spoken or written words.
c. <**A**nomic aphasia occurs in lesions of **A**ngular gyrus>

There is trouble in understanding written languages and pictures. Patient cannot name objects.
See Fig. 3.8.

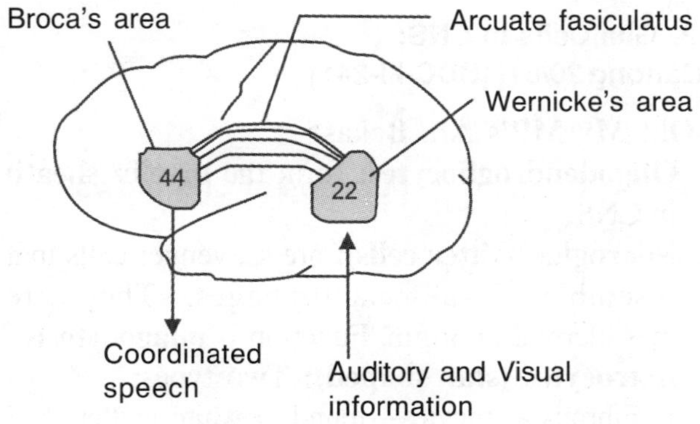

Fig. 3.8

17. Cerebellar Deep Nuclei

<**L**adies **D**emand **E**xceptional **G**enerosity **F**rom **M**en>:

The 4 nuclei, from lateral to medial:
[**L**ateral]
Dentate
Emboliform
Globose
Fastigial
[**M**edial]

Or simply remember: **<DEFG>**

18. Cerebellar Functional Areas

Anatomical shape/location of cerebellar areas is a key to their function and related tract.

a. Spinocerebellum = Vermis = Posture of limbs and skilled voluntary movements.
   It lies along the axis and is segmented like the spinal cord.
b. Vestibulocerebellum = Flocculonodular lobe = Ear, eye, body coordination.
   It flares out to the edges, just like ears.
c. Cerebrocerebellum =Hemispheres of cerebellum = Planning and modulation.
   It lies around periphery of cerebellum, and receives input from cerebral hemispheres.

See Fig. 3.9 and Table 3.1.

19. Glia Cells in CNS: [Ganong 20/61] [BDC-III-241]

<**O**h! **M**y **MP**'s **A**re **B**okas>

1. **Oligodendrogliocytes:** form the **myelin sheath** in CNS.
2. **Microglia (Gitter cells):** are scavenger cells that resemble tissue macrophages. They are mesodermal in origin. Function is **phagocytosis.**
3. **Astrocytes (star shaped):** Two types:
   i. Fibrous astrocytes—found in white matter,

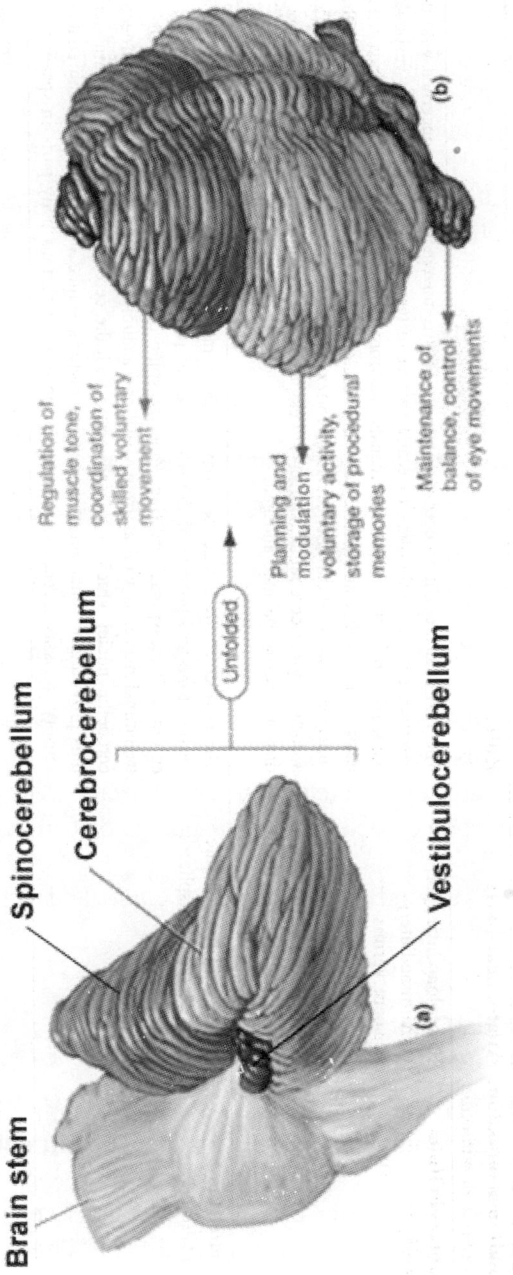
Brain stem
Spinocerebellum
Cerebrocerebellum
Vestibulocerebellum
(a)
Unfolded
Regulation of muscle tone, coordination of skilled voluntary movement
Planning and modulation voluntary activity, storage of procedural memories
Maintenance of balance, control of eye movements
(b)

Fig. 3.9

Table 3.1

Functional denomination *(phylogenetic denomination)*	**Anatomical parts**	**Role**
Vestibulocerebellum *(Archicerebellum)*	Flocculonodular lobe (and immediately adjacent vermis	The vestibulocerebellum regulates balance and eye movements. It is concerned with the maintainence of equilibrium, tone and posture of trunk muscles. It receives vestibular input from both the semicircular canals and from the vestibular nuclei, and sends fibres back to the medial and lateral vestibular nuclei. It also receives visual input from the superior colliculi and from the visual cortex (the latter via the pontine nuclei, forming a cortico-ponto-cerebellar pathway). Lesions of the vestibulocerebellum cause disturbances of balance and gait.
Spinocerebellum *(Paleocerebellum)*	Vermis and intermediate parts of the hemispheres ("paravermis")	The spinocerebellum regulates body and limb movements. It has got significant role in muscle tone and posture of limbs. It receives proprioception input from the dorsal columns of the spinal cord (including the spinocerebellar tract) as well as from the trigeminal nerve, as well as from visual and auditory systems. It sends fibres to deep cerebellar nuclei which in turn project to both the cerebral cortex and the brain stem, thus providing modulation of descending motor systems. The spinocerebellum contains sensory maps as it receives data on the position of various body parts in space: in

Contd.

Contd.

		particular, the vermis receives fibres from the trunk and proximal portions of limbs, while the intermediate parts of the hemispheres receive fibres from the distal portions of limbs. The spinocerebellum is able to elaborate proprioceptive input in order to anticipate the future position of a body part during the course of a movement, in a "feed forward" manner.
Cerebrocerebellum *(Neocerebellum, Pontocerebellum)*	Lateral parts of the hemispheres	The neocerebellum is involved in planning movement and evaluating sensory information for action. It receives input exclusively from the cerebral cortex (especially the parietal lobe) via the pontine nuclei (forming cortico-ponto-cerebellar pathways), and sends fibres mainly to the ventrolateral thalamus (in turn connected to motor areas of the premotor cortex and primary motor area of the cerebral cortex) and to the red nucleus (in turn connected to the inferior olivary nucleus, which links back to the cerebellar hemispheres). The neocerebellum is involved in planning movement that is about to occur and has purely cognitive functions as well.

ii. Protoplasmic astrocytes—found in gray matter.**Astrocytes form the Blood-brain-barrier**

☑ Schwann cells form the myelin sheath in PNS

20. Cerebellum: Functional Divisions [BDC-III-265]

<**P**oor **S**abrina **C**an **N**ever **C**hat **P**ublicly with **A**rchi **V**eronica & **B**etty>

Division	*Alternate name*	*Function*
Paleocerebellum	**S**pinocerebellum	**C**oordination
Neocerebellum	**C**erebrocerebellum	**P**lanning
Archicerebellum	**V**estibulocerebellum	**B**alance

Alternatively (In Hindi):
<**P**yari **S**abrina **C**o, **A**rchi **V**eronica & **B**etty, **N**e **C**hot **P**ahuchai>

21. Relative Susceptibility of Nerve Fibers: [Ganong 20th-59]

Susceptibility to	*Most susceptible*	*Intermediate*	*Least susceptible*
Hypoxia	**B**	**A**	**C**
Pressure	**A**	B	C
Local anesthetic	**C**	B	A

Mnemonic: <**HPL = BAC / BAC**>

Another one: **OBC / PAC / LOCA**
OBC
O- oxygen (Hypoxia)
B – Most susceptible
C – Least susceptible

PAC
P- pressure
A – Most susceptible
C – Least susceptible

LOCA
LO – local anesthetic
C- Most susceptible
A – Least susceptible

22. Circumventricular Organs: [Ganong 20th Ed/P-592]

These areas have fenestrated capillaries and because of their permeability are said to be outside the blood brain barrier (BBB).
Mnemonic: <**SOAP**>

1. **S**ubforniceal organ (SFO)
2. **O**rganum vasculosum of the lamina terminalis (OVLT, supraoptic crest)
3. **A**rea postrema
4. **P**osterior pituitary (neurohypophysis) and the adjacent ventral part of the median eminence of hypothalamus.

Functions of each these organs:

1. SFO—Angiotensin II acts here to increase water intake.
2. OVLT—It is the site for osmoreceptor controlling vasopressin secretion.
3. Area postrema—It has the chemoreceptor trigger zone (CTZ) which initiates vomiting. It is also concerned with cardiovascular control
4. Posterior pituitary—(neurohemal organ) – Oxytocin and vasopressin enter the general circulation here.
5. Median eminence of the hypothalamus—(neurohemal organ) – Hypothalamic and pituitary regulatory hormones enter the portal hypophysial circulation here from the general circulation.

☑ *The pineal gland and anterior pituitary also have fenestrated capillaries and are outside the blood brain barrier, but both of them are endocrine glands and are not part of the brain.*
— Ganong 20th Ed/P-593

23. Conduction Speed in Cardiac Tissue: [Ganong 20th Ed/P-530]

Tissue	*Conduction rate (m/s)*
SA node	0.05
AV node	0.05
Bundle of His	1
Atrial pathways	1
Ventricular pathways	1
Purkinje system	4

Mnemonic:
1. **Nodes** look like nodes— 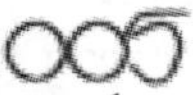
2. **His atria** and **ventricles** are 1
3. Purkinje = **Fourkinje** = 4

24. Lower vs. Upper Motor Neuron Lesion Effects

1. **<STORM Baby>**
   STORM Baby tells you effects:
   - **S**trength
   - **T**one
   - **O**ther
   - **R**eflexes
   - **M**uscle mass
   - **Bab**inski's sign.
2. **<In a Lower motor neuron lesion, everything goes Down:>**
   Strength, tone, reflexes, muscle mass, and the big toe is down in plantar reflex (Babinski's sign is negative)

25. Effects of Lesion of Pyramidal Tract (Upper Motor Neuron) [BDC-III-294]

<Pyramid BLASTS>
B—**B**abinski sign positive
L—**L**oss of voluntary movements
A—**A**bsent reaction of degeneration
S—**S**uperficial reflexes are lost
T—**T**endon reflexes are exaggerated
S—**S**pastic Paralysis (Clasp-Knife type)

26. Babinski's Sign : Upper Motor vs. Lower Motor Neuron Lesion

<Toe **UP**>

Toe is **U**p (Planter reflex – extensor) in **U**MLN and is called Babinski's **P**ositive.

27. Olivary Nuclei: Ear vs. Eye Roles

<**S**uperior **O**livary nucleus: **SO**und localization>.
Inferior olivary nucleus is therefore the one for sight [tactile, proprioception also].

28. Bell-Magendie Law: [ganong 20th- 123]

The principle that in the spinal cord dorsal roots are sensory and the ventral roots are motor is known as the Bell-**MA**gendie law.

<**MA** : **M**otor is **A**nterior>

29. Precentral vs. Postcentral Gyrus: Motor vs. Sensory

Just an extension of the above rule that **anterior = ventral = efferent = motor**.

The precentral gyrus is on the anterior side of the central sulcus, so is therefore motor.

The postcentral gyrus is on the posterior side of the central sulcus, so is therefore sensory.

30. Pathway of Light Reflex: [BDC-III-297, Khurana 3rd Ed/P-279]

<**R**atna **O**beys **O**rders **O**f **La**zy **P**rince **E**dinger's **3** Children>

Retina
Optic nerve
Optic chaiasma
Optic tract
Lateral geniculate body
Pretectal nucleus
Edinger-Westphal nucleus
3rd cranial nerve

3C's – **C**iliary ganglion
short **C**iliary nerve
Constrictor pupilae

Old Menmonic:
<**R**amu **O**nly **O**beys **O**rders to **L**ate **P**rince **E**dinger & **3 C**hildren>

☑ To remember that the ciliary nerve is 'short' think of children who are 'small'.

31. Pathway of Accommodation Reflex: [BDC-III-297, Khurana 3rd -279]

<**R**atna **A**lways **O**beys **O**ut **O**f **LOVeS** *for* **E**dinger's **3 C**hildren>

Retina
[**A**ccomodation]
Optic nerve
Optic chaiasma
Optic tract
Lateral geniculate body
Optic radiation
Visual cortex
Superior longitudinal association tract
Edinger-Westphal nucleus
3rd cranial nerve
3C's – **C**iliary ganglion
Ciliary muscle
Constrictor pupilae

Old Menmonic:
<**R**amu **O**nly **O**beys **O**rders **L**ately **O**n **V**eryfing **S**ervice **F**or **E**dinger's **3 C**hildren>

32. Triple Response: [Ganong 22nd – 625] [SKC-262]

Triple response or Axon Reflex: When an area of skin is stroked, sensory nerve fibers, arising from the area are stimulated and carry the impulse to the respective spinal cord segments as usual. However during this journey, a branch of this nerve gets activated and the impulse returns back to a cutaneous arteriole (without reaching the spinal cord) causing this arteriole to dilate. This is one of the few reflexes in our body which does not involve the CNS. This is also the reason why triple response is intact even after total sympathetectomy.

When the skin is stroked very firmly, by the smooth end of a stick or a glass rod the characteristic triple response develops: Its features are:

1. Red line—due to **H**istamine release which causes relaxation of pericapillary sphincter which in turn causes capillary engorgement.
2. **F**lare—due to **A**xonal reflex which causes arteriolar dilatation beyond the stroked area.
3. **W**heal—due to **E**deme fluid collection which transudates from the engorged capillaries.

Mnemonic : <**R**ed **H**ot **F**emales **A**lways **W**ant **E**rotic **T**ools>

The last '**T**' helps you to remember that this mnemonic is for **Triple response**.

☑ *Also know*: Some people are very sensitive, so much so, that a moderate or even mild stroking produces an exaggerated triple response on their skin. This phenomenon is called *dermographism.* Dermographism is seen in urticaria.

33. Photochemistry of Vision: [SKC-587] [Ganong-22nd-158]

"Once upon a time a fat boy called 'Alene' was standing on the roof and enjoying the cool breeze with both his hands up. Suddenly lightning struck him in one hand and his hand was broken. Poor 'Alene' was so fat that he could not be carried in one piece so it was decided to leave behind ½ his body. He was taken to the dark and mysterious Wizard who repaired his arm and did some magic to rejoin both halves of his body. Fat Alene was once again happily enjoying the cool breeze when lightning struck him again…" See Fig. 3.10a.

- The word **'<u>Alene</u>'** comes from 'Retin**<u>al</u>** and Retin**<u>ene</u>**' both of which are one and the same thing.
- The fat part of his body is **Scotopsin.**
- Alene is the Rhodopsin (Rhodopsin = Scotopsin + Retinal)
- Conversion of all-cis retinal to all-trans retinal helps in the amplification of light signal by activating a protein called transducin which in turn activates cGMP.
- The dark wizard is Retinal Isomerase.
- New all-cis-retinal can be generated from vit. A (all-trans-retinol). See Fig. 3.10b.

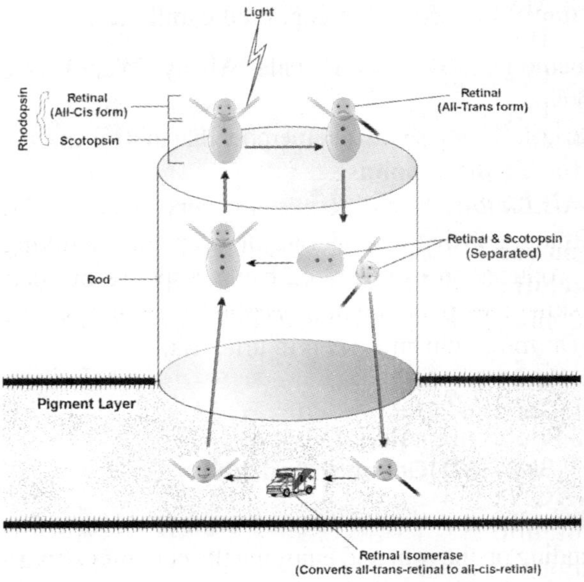

Fig. 3.10a: Neurophysiology of vision

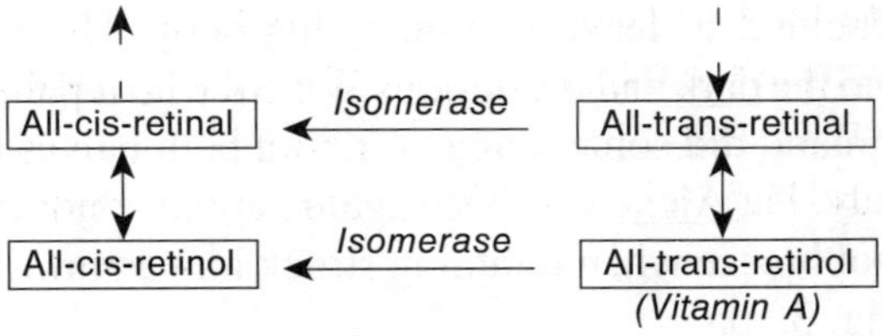

Fig. 3.10b

34. Colour Blindness: [Ganong 22nd Ed/P-164]

Mnemonic *(in Hindi)*
<**B**ombay **T**o **G**oa **D**o **R**upiya **P**achas *paisa*>
Blue blindness – **T**ritanopia
Green blindness – **D**uteranopia
Red blindness – **P**rotanopia

☑ *Also Remember:*

- The suffix '–anomaly' means colour weakness and the '-anopia' means complete colour blindness.
- Dichromats can see only 2 colours
- Monochromats can see only 1 colour
- Most common type of colour blindness is **Duteranomaly** (green).
- Colour blindness is X-linked recessive
- Primary visual cortex is V_1 area.
- Colour vision cortex is V_8 area.

35. C- fibers (nerves): [Ganong 22nd – 61]

<You can C (see) the naked C-fibers as it wears no clothes.>
☑ C-fibers are unmyelinated fibers.

36. Neurotransmitters: [Ganong 22nd Ed/P-107, 20th Ed/P-92]

Two most important neurotransmitters in CNS are:
<GAGA>
Glutamic **A**cid (glutamate)– Main excitatory neurotransmitter (75%).
GABA – Main inhibitory neurotransmitter.

Other important ones:

- Aspartate is excitatory neurotransmitter
- Glycine is inhibitory
- Acetylcholine
- Two gases act as neurotransmitter in brain: NO and CO.

Amine neurotransmitters are:
<DiNESH>
- **D**opamine
- **N**orepinephrine
- **E**pinephrine
- **S**erotonine
- **H**istamine

36. Role of Substance P:

<Substance **P** is **P**ain producing Substance >

IV. RESPIRATION

1. Factors Affecting Compliance of Lungs [G-656]

<COMPLIANCE>

Collagen deposition (fibrosis)
Ossification of costal cartilages
Major obesity
Pulmonary venous congestion
Lung size*
Increased expanding pressure
Age*
No surfactant
Chest wall scarring
Emphysema*
* *All but L/A/E decrease compliance.*
L/A/E increase compliance

2. Ventilation and Perfusion of Lungs:

<BAD Ventilation & Perfusion>

Base to **A**pex **D**ecreases — **V**entilation and **P**erfusion. Both Ventilation and Perfusion are more at the base than at the apex.

☑ Remember V/Q and PaO_2 is more at the apex than at the base.

3. Lung Surfactant:

Count the no. of letters in <Surfactant production> you will get the no. of weeks

☑ Surfactant production starts in **20** weeks of life.
☑ It peaks at 35 weeks.
☑ Neonates less than 35 weeks are prone to develop 'Respiratory Distress Syndrome'

4. Respiratory Centers: [SKC- 156]

☑ They are located in **medulla.**
☑ There are **two groups** of these respiratory neurons.

i. **Ventral group**: This is a long column of neurons, present in ventrolateral part of medulla from Nucleus ambigualis to Nucleus retroambigualis region.
It has mainly **E neuron** (expiratory) at the rostral and caudal end and some **I neurons** (inspiratory) at the middle part.

ii. **Dorsal group** : It is located **in** and **near** Nucleus tractus solitarius. It has mainly **I neurons.**

Mnemonic:

InSpiratory centre à DorSal
Expiratory centre à VEntral

Remember:

☑ The I neurons are firing all the time and the E neurons do not fire in the normal quiet breathing.
☑ Pre Botzing complex is the Pacemaker.
See Fig 3.11.

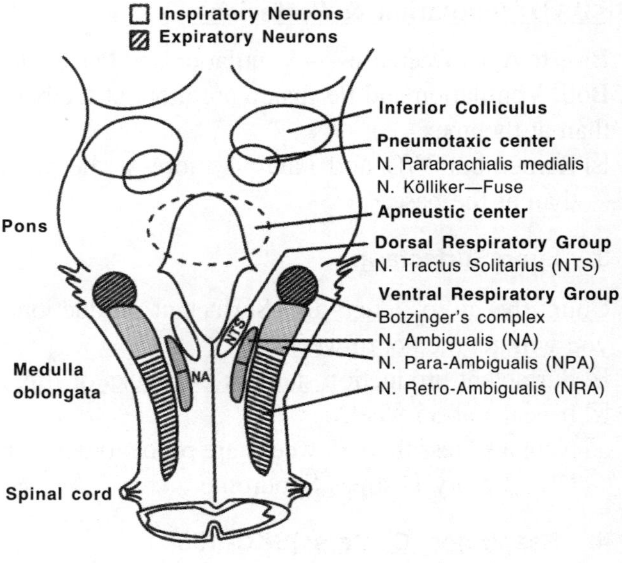

Fig. 3.11

5. <u>Two Types of Beta Receptors are</u>

β_1 = You have one heart so found in heart.
β_2 = you have two lungs so found in the bronchi.

6. <u>Hypoxia: Vascular Changes</u> [Ganong 20th Ed/P-641]

<Blood goes to the lungs to take oxygen: So if there is no oxygen in lungs why will blood go there ?>
<Blood goes to the rest of body's tissues to give oxygen: So if there is no oxygen in the tissues more blood will go there to give more oxygen.>

Therefore hypoxia causes vasodilatation in all tissues except lungs where it causes vasoconstriction.

7. <u>Diffusion Capacity of Lungs</u> [Ganong 20th Ed/P-638]

Diffusion **C**apacity **O**f **L**ungs:
Rearrange the first letter of each word and you get DLCO (DL_{CO}).

So diffusion capacity of lungs is measured by diffusion capacity of Carbon Monoxide.
***Normal DL_{CO} at rest is about **25ml/min/mmHg.**

8. <u>Hypoxia</u> [Ganong 20th Ed/P-660]

Four important steps are required for the transport of oxygen to the tissues:
1. Loading of oxygen in the lungs
2. Hemoglobin
3. Circulation
4. Unloading in the tissue.

There are four types of hypoxia:
Mnemonic: "**HASH**".

	Type	*Basic defect in*	*Reduction in*	*Example*
1.	**H**ypoxic hypoxia	Loading of oxygen in the lungs	PaO_2 in arterial blood	Lung diseases, cyanotic congenital heart diseases, cystic fibrosis
2.	**A**nemic hypoxia	Hemoglobin	O_2 carrying capacity of	Severe anemia, CO poisoning

		blood	
3. **S**tagnant hypoxia	Circulation	Rate of blood flow	Congestive heart failure, shock
4. **H**istotoxic hypoxia	Unloading in the tissue	Utilization of O_2 in tissues	Cyanide poisoning

Also know:

☑ Cyanosis is absent in anemic hypoxia, carbon monoxide poisoning and in histotoxic hypoxia.

☑ Hypoxia is a potent vasodilator in all body tissues except lungs where it constricts pulmonary arteries.

☑ A normal individual is not conscious of respiration until ventilation is doubled.

☑ Breathing is not uncomfortable (i.e. dyspnea point is not reached) until ventilation is tripled or quadrupled.

☑ Dyspneic index is the percentage of respiratory capacity not being used at a given respiratory minute volume. When the dyspneic index is less than about 70%, dyspnea is usually present.

V. MISCELLANEOUS

1. Cell Cycle

"**G**o **S**ally **G**o! **M**ake **C**hildren."
G1, S, G2, M, C

- **G**rowth phase 1
- DNA **S**ynthesis (replication)
- **G**rowth phase 2
- **M**itosis
- **C**ytokinesis.

2. Mitosis

<**P**eople **M**eet **A**nd **T**alk> or <**PMAT**>
Prophase, Metaphase, Anaphase, Telophase.

3. Meiosis

<PMAT x2>
Prophase I, Metaphase I, Anaphase I, Telophase I, Prophase II, Metaphase II, Anaphase II, Telophase II.

(*Note:* Four haploid daughter cells instead of 2 diploid daughter cells).

4. Immunoglobulins

<GAMED>
IgG
IgA
IgM
IgE
IgD.

5. Total Body Water [Ganong-20th Ed/P_1, 2]

1. "**I**CF and **I**nterstitial fluid volume are **I**mpossible to measure directly."
2. "**H_2O** is measured by **D_2O**"—(Total body water is measured by using D_2O).
3. **Plasma volume**—measured by <u>Albumin</u> tagged by radioactive iodine or <u>Evan's blue dye</u>.

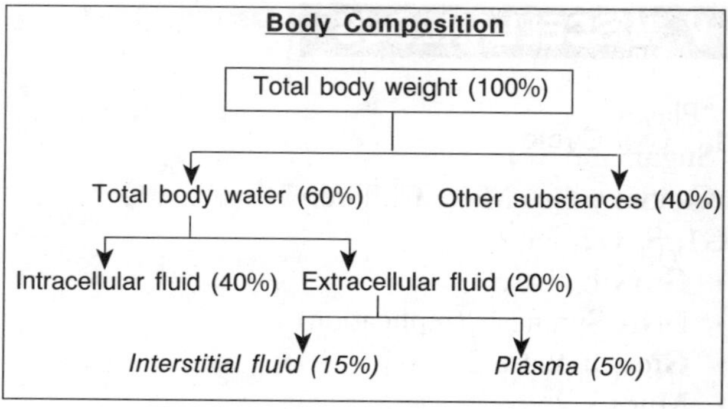

Fig. 3.12: Body composition

4. **RBC volume**—measured by **Cr^{51}-tagged RBC.**
5. **ECF volume**—measured by sugars such as inulin, mannitol, sucrose etc. (**Inulin** is the best indicator among these.)

☑ Total body water is:

- Somewhat lower in women
- Tends to decrease with age
- Lesser in fatty persons.

☑ Lean body mass = Body mass devoid of fat.

6. Osmolarity vs. Osmolality [Ganong 20th—5]

Osmolarity is no. of osmotically active particles in 1 liter of the solution (mOsm/L).

Osmolality is no. of osmotically active particles in 1 Kg of the solution (mOsm/Kg).

Osmolarity is affected by variations in the volume of various solutes in the solution and the temperature, whereas osmolality is not. Therefore osmolality is a better measurement than osmolarity.

Mnemonic: "osmola**R**ity = lit**R**e = affected by va**R**iations".

☑ Freezing point of normal human plasma = **-0.54°C**

☑ Normal plasma osmolality = **290 mosm/L.**

7. How to Calculate Plasma Osmolality [Ganong 22nd Ed/P-6]

"Plasma osmolality is nothing but **a BUN with some Sugar and Salt**".

Ganong gives the formula of plasma osmolality as:

$$\text{Osmolality} = 2[Na^+]_{\text{mEq/L}} + 0.055[\text{Glucuse}]_{\text{mg/dL}} + 0.36[\text{BUN}]_{\text{mg/dL}}$$

Not only is this formula difficult to remember but it is also very difficult to do any calculation with it.

The same formula can be written in a much simpler way:

$$\text{Osmolality} = 2[Na^+]_{\text{(mEq/L)}} + \frac{10}{180}[\text{Glucuse}]_{\text{(mg/dL)}} + \frac{10}{28}[\text{BUN}]_{\text{mg/dL}}$$

If you see carefully, the formula is nothing but the sum of osmolality of the three substances.

If you are still not convinced let's see how it is derived:

Facts:

Molecular weight: Glucose = 180 , BUN = 28

1 mEq/L of Na^+ = 1 mOsm/L of Na^+

1 mg/dL of Glucose = 10 mg/L = 10/180 mOsm/L of glucose = 0.055 mOsm/L of glucose

1 mg/dL of BUN = 10 mg/L = 10/28 mOsm/L of BUN = 0.36 mOsm/L of BUN.

Na^+, glucose and BUN are the major contributors of plasma osmolality. Na^+ is taken twice because the Na^+ ion is always associated with a cation (chloride or bicarbonate) which itself will contribute to the plasma osmolality. Since the no. of cations will balance the no. of sodium ions we do not need to know the exact no. of cations.

*** *Note:* If a question gives plasma values of other substances as well, then you have to calculate the osmolality of each of them and then add them up to get the total osmolality.

8. Molecular Weight of Some Common Substances in Medicine**

Hydrogen–H–1
Carbon–C–12
Oxygen–O–16
Sodium—Na—23
Chloride—Cl—35.5
Potassium—K—39
Calcium—Ca—40
Sulphur—S—32
Glucose—180
Urea/BUN—28
** Sorry no mnemonic for this.

9. Anion Gap [Ganong 20th Ed/P-710]

Routine serum electrolyte determination measures most of the cations but only a few anions. This apparent disparity between the total cation and the total anion concentration is called the anion gap.

Anion gap = [(Na+) + (K+)] - [(Cl^-) + (HCO^-)] = normally about 10-16 mmol/L (average 12).
Mnemonic: [All plus ions]–[All minus ions].

10. The Mathematics of $Na^{\pm}$ and $K^{\pm}$ ions [Ganong 22nd Ed/P-8]

<Potassium = Cytoplasm= 9>
<Sodium = Plasma= 6>

Count the letters in each word: So potassium is more abundant in the cytoplasm and sodium is more in plasma.

Na^+-K^+ ATPase:
<HIKIN>
There is a **HI**gh **K** concentration **IN**side the cell.

From this can deduce that the Na^+/K^+ pump pumps K+ into cell and Na+ out of cell.

<Potassium + Potassium = 18>
<Sodium + Sodium + Sodium =18>

Therefore: Na^+ K^+ ATPase transfers $2K^+$ into the cell and $3Na^+$ out of the cell.

It can also be remembered as:

K+ and in each consist of 2 characters, so so 2 K+ are pumped in.

Na+ and out each consist of 3 characters, so 3 Na+ are pumped out.

☑ **M**embrane **P**otential is due to **P**otassiu**M**.

☑ **Pacemaker** potential is due to decrease in **Potassium** efflux.

☑ Actio**N** potential is due to Sodium (**Na**).

11. Apoptosis: Role of Caspases [Ganong 22nd Ed/P-26]

<Casp-Ase> = **<Gasp-Age>**
'Casp' rhymes with 'Gasp'
'Ase' rhymes with 'Age'.

Think of a cell that is dying of old age and gasping in its last times.

Apoptosis means programmed cell death i.e. A cell dies its natural death when it reaches its biological old age. The final common pathway bringing about apoptosis is the activation of caspases, a group of cysteine proteases. The net result is DNA fragmentation, cytoplasmic and chromatin condensation and eventually membrane bleb formation, with cell breakup and removal of debris by phagocytes.

*** *Note:* There is no inflammatory process involved unlike necrosis.

12. Chaperones: Role in Protein Folding [Harper 26th Ed/P-507] [Ganong 22nd Ed/P-25]

<Chaper-ones> (Read as cheaper ones).

Since our body could not afford costly machines for folding proteins it went for "Cheaper ones"!

"In some instances, nascent proteins associate with other proteins called chaper ones, which prevent inappropriate contact with other proteins and ensure that the final proper conformation of the nascent protein is reached."—Ganong.

13. Ubiquitin: Role in Protein Degradation [Ganong 21st Ed/P-507] [Ganong 22nd Ed/P-297, 25]

<U' be quitting!>

Ubiquitin says to the intracellular proteins—"U be quitting!"

Means that the protein has to quit its job and get degraded.

"Aged and misfolded proteins are conjugated with 74-aminoacid polypeptide ubiquitin, which ticks them for degradation. These proteins are then degraded by multisubunit proteolytic particles, the **26S proteosomes**."—Ganong

14. Clathrin: Role in Endocytosis [Ganong 22nd Ed/P-28,29]

<Clathrin likes **"Clear and Thin"** (i.e. water)>
Clathrin helps in pinocytosis and phagocytosis (Clathrin mediated endocytosis).

15. Balance Organs in Ear [G-173]

"**U** **H**ave **S**ymptoms of **V**ertigo".
Utricle = Horizontal acceleration.
Saccule = Vertical acceleration.

Semi**circular** canal = **Circular** (rotational) accleration.

16. Barr Body [Rudolph's Textbook of Pediatrics 21st Ed]

<InterSex are Barred>
Barr body is **X** chromosome in **Interphase**.

- **The two X-chrmosomes in females diploid somatic cells exhibit striking morphologic and functional differences:**
  1. **One X-chromosome is in a highly condensed (Heteropyknotic) state in INTERPHASE and is visible as sex chromatin (BARR BODY).** It completes DNA synthesis later than any other chromosome, and the **action**

of genes located on the precociously condensed segments is suppressed by transcriptional inactivation.

2. **The other X-chromosome,** the single X-chromosome in male somatic cells, is in a highly extended (isopyknotic) state during INTERPHASE. It completes DNA replication with most of the complement and is **genetically active.**

- The discordant behavior of two homologous X-chromosomes in female somatic cells serves as a mechanism of dosage compensation.

17. Alcohol: Energy Production

< **Alcohol** has **7** letters so it gives **7**cal/gm of energy>

18. Intercellular Connections [Ganong 20th Ed/P16] [AKD-General Anatomy-39]

1. **Gap junctions:**
   Gap—Gaps in the cell membrane .
   Junction—Neighboring cells are joined by **Connexons.**
   Gap junctions allow substances to pass between the cells without entering the ECF.

☑ *Diseases linked to mutant connexons:*
- Charcot-Marie-Tooth disease.
- Heterotaxia.

2. **Tight junctions:**
   Tight junctions are **water tight** and **pack the cells tightly**.
   Found in apical margins of epithelial cells in intestinal mucosa, choroid plexus, renal tubules, etc.
   Prevent passage of ions and solutes in between the cells.
   Also called Zona Occludens.
3. **Desmosomes and hemidesmosomes:**
   In desmosomes the inner lamina of each cell membrane is **dense** (thickened).

Contains intermediate filaments running parallel to the cell membranes.

Many transmembrane proteins are present in the desmosomes.

Hemidesmosomes look like half desmosomes and are present between the cell basement membrane.

19. Golgi Apparatus [Ganong 20th Ed/P-26,27] [AKD-General Anatomy—23]

Cis golgi—Collects vesicles from rough endoplasmic reticulum.

Trans golgi—Transports vesicles to lysosomes and secretory vesicles.

The golgi apparatus is a polarized structure with cis and trans sides. It works like a "**post office**" for proteins. Proteins are received by the cis face of the Golgi and exit through the trans face after modification.

Other functions: <**MAST**>

- **M**odification of carbohydrate attached to glycoproteins.
- **A**ddition of mannose to proteins destined for lysosomes.
- **S**ecretion of glycocalyx (cell-coat) in non-secretory cells.
- **T**emporary storage of hormones and enzymes until released (thus protecting the cells from its own enzymes).

20. Osteoblast vs. Osteoclast [G-387]

Osteo**B**last **B**uilds bone.

Osteo**C**last **C**onsumes bone.

21. Digestive Juices:

☑ **Bile** Breaks fat into Blobs.

☑ Chief stomach enzyme is **Pepsin** ... remember drinking **Pepsi** to help his digestion.

☑ **Parietal** cells: **P**roduce **A**cid, **R**elease **I**ntrinsic factor, **ET AL**.

22. Causes of Blood in the Urine:

The six common causes of blood in the urine:
<SHITTT>
Stones
Hematological Disorder
Infection
Tumor
Tuberculosis
Trauma

23. 8 functions of blood:

<Waste Ox Carried Diseased Food making **Clot in Heated Whore>**

Waste
Oxygen
Carbon dioxide
Disease
Food
Clotting
Heat
Hormones

☑ Of course, I related the hormones to "whore moans".

24. Quick Blood/Cardio Facts

☑ **Tricuspid** valve is in The Right Inside part of the heart.
☑ **Mitral** is on Left side.
☑ **B** Cells Bite virus, **T** Cells Torpedo sick cells.
☑ Remember **Lying Nude in Basement Early Monday** has every white blood cell mentioned: Lymphocytes, Neutrophils, Basophils, Eosinophils, and Monocytes.

25. Centrioles

Centrioles are useful organelles which play a key role in cell division, namely pulling the chromosomes apart.

Centrioles are ropes made of 9 groups of 3 fibres, a **9+3** arrangement. How to remember this? Count the number of letters in "centriole", then count the syllables. You should get 9 and 3.

26. Mitosis

<I Proposed Marriage to Anna by Telephone before I Sighted her Cleavage>

Interphase
Prophase
Metaphase
Anaphase
Telophase
Cytokinesis (sighted) and
cell **C**leavage

27. Mitosis and Meiosis

Easy way to tell the difference between the two types of reproduction at the cell level:
Mitosis makes Identical Twins
Meiosis makes Egg and Sperm.

28. Hormones : Quick Facts

☑ 8 major hormones from the pituitary gland spell **GOAT-FLAP**: gonadotropic, oxytocin, anti-diuretic, thyroid stimulating, follicle stimulating, leuteinizing, adrenocorticotropic, prolactin.

☑ The pituitary gland has two lobes: anterior and posterior. 6 of the preceding hormones come from the anterior lobe; oxytocin and anti-diuretic are secreted from the posterior one.

☑ The adrenal **CORTex** produces **CORTisol**, as well as androgens and aldosterone.

☑ The adrenal Medulla secretes stress hormones Epinephrine and Norepinephrine and, as all women know, men are a source of stress, so it is no surprise that medulla-epinephrine-norepinephrine make the acronym **MEN**.

☑ Adrenal Cortex hormones start with either of letters **A, C** — just like adrenal cortex. They are: androgen, aldosterone, cortisol.

☑ Ovaries are **RIPE** with hormones: relaxin, inhibin, progesterone, estrogen make the acronym RIPE.

☑ Testes make **TIM** strong: "t.i.m." is acronym for the 3 hormones secreted by testes: testosterone, inhibin, and Mullerian-inhibiting hormones.

☑ Pancreas makes **PIGS**: Pancreatic polypeptide, Insulin, Glucagon, and Somatostatin hormones.

☑ **Some Secret Gas Choked GIPsy** represents the 5 hormones of the (where do you think gas comes from?) gastrointestinal tract: somatostatin, secretin, gastrin, cholecystokinin, glucose-dependent insulinotropic peptide (GIP).

☑ Melatonin makes penis pineal? **Melatonin** secreted from pineal gland represses sex drive.

☑ A **Hypocritical Gun-Running Hero goes to Pit to release Long Hard Fish, but is turned off the the smell of Estrogen**. That was the story of the hypothalamus secreting GnRH (Gun-running hero) to stimulate the Pituitary gland into releasing LH and FSH. This process is regulated by the levels of estrogen.

☑ Products of the adrenal cortex, from outer to inner layer: "**Salt, sugar, sex; It gets sweeter as you get deeper**" (Salt=aldosterone, sugar= glucocorticoids, sex=sex hormones).

MULTIPLE CHOICE QUESTIONS

1. **Given EEG is suggestive of:**

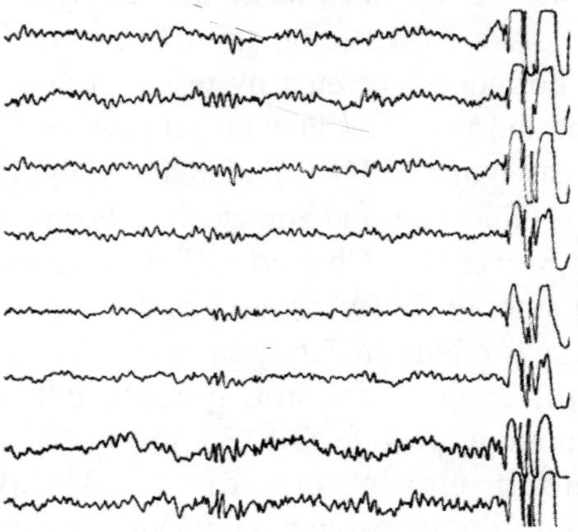

A. Bifrontal spike and wave
B. Movement artifact
C. Polyspike and wave
D. Generalized slow spike and wave

2. **Sympathetic stimulation increases blood flow to all except:**

A. Skin
B. Coronary circulation
C. Cerebral
D. Renal

3. **All of the following are true about excitation contraction coupling except:**

A. Acetylcholine is released at the nerve terminal
B. Calcium is pumped back into the sarcoplasmic reticulum during relaxation
C. Calcium is released from sarcoplasmic reticulum during contraction
D. Calcium binds to tropomyosin to initiate muscle contraction

4. **Transcutaneous electrical nerve stimulation based on:**

A. Central pain
B. Referred pain
C. Gate controlled theory of pain
D. Allodynia

5. All of the following are rue about Kluver-Bucy syndrome expect:
A. Hypersexuality
B. Hyperactivity
C. Hypermetamorphosis
D. Placidity

6. Peripheral resistance is best indicated by:
A. Diastolic blood pressure
B. Pulse pressure
C. Systolic resistance in aorta as it increases in its length
D. Mean arterial pressure, which is responsible for blood flow to an organ

7. Blood testis barrier is located between:
A. Sertoli and sertoli cells
B. Leydig and myoid cells
C. Sertoli and germ cells
D. Sertoli spermatid

8. Release of synaptic vesicle from presynaptic terminal is inhibited by:
A. Stopping action potential
B. Prevention of Na+ influx
C. Prevention of Ca2+ influx
D. Stop depolarisation

9. What happens immediately after lying down?
A. Increase in cerebral blood flow
B. Immediately increase in venous return to heart
C. Decreased blood flow to lung apex
D. Increase in heart rate

10. Which of the following statement is true regarding time of ovulation?
A. Occurs before LH surge
B. Occurs after biphasic rise in basal body temperature
C. Occurs after follicular ripening by FSH
D. Occurs after disappearance of cervical mucus thickening

11. Neuroendocrine cells in the lumen of the tracheobronchial tree:
A. Contain serotonin
B. Contain catecholamines
C. Respond to decrease in pO2
D. Have only cholinergic nerve supply

12. Fick's law (Flick's law was in given in the paper):
A. For passive diffusion down the concentration gradient
B. Passive osmosis along concentration gradient
C. Active osmosis along concentration gradient
D. Active and passive movement of molecule along concentration gradient

13. Embryonal hemoglobin is formed by:
A. Epsilon and zeta
B. Epsilon and gamma
C. Alpha and delta
D. Beta and gamma

14. All of the following are true about Kluver-Bucy syndrome except:
A. Visual agnosia
B. Hypersexuality
C. Hypermetamorphosis
D. Intractable seizures

15. A motorcyclist after road traffic accident is having raised arterial pCO2 on ABG. Probable cause can be:
A. Damage to respiratory apparatus
B. Damage to respiratory centre
C. Damage to both respiratory apparatus and respiratory centre
D. Massive lung contusion alone

16. Biomineralization is a process by which inorganic "metals" are incorporated in the body and made a part of biological structures. Example of Biomineralization is seen in:
A. Pinna (anatomy)
B. Hooves of cattle
C. Honeycomb
D. Mollusc shell

17. Following microinjection to cell membrane, healing occurs by:
A. Lateral movement of proteins
B. ATP dependent enzyme activity
C. Hydrophobic interactions
D. Energy dependent active process

18. While seeing a colour chart a colour blind male has decreased vision for red light colour which appear very light than that of other colours. Which of the following is the likely anomaly in him?

A. Protanomaly
B. Dutanomaly
C. Tritanomaly
D. Butanomaly

19. The pacemaker potential is due to:

A. Fast Na^{+}channel
B. Decrease in K^{+} permeability
C. Slow Ca^{++} channel
D. Rapid repolarization

20. How much amount of energy is yielded by one ml of alcohol in the body?

A. 1 cal
B. 4 cal
C. 7 cal
D. 9 cal

21. During acclimatization to high altitude all of the following take place *except*:

A. Increase in minute ventilation
B. Increase in the sensitivity of central chemoreceptors
C. Increase in the sensitivity of carotid body to hypoxia
D. Shift in the oxygen dissociation curve to the left

22. The main excitatory neurotransmitter in the CNS is:

A. Glycine
B. Acetylcholine
C. Aspartate
D. Glutamate

23. Proteins targeted for destruction in eukaryotes are covalently linked to:

A. Clathrin
B. Pepsin

C. Laminin
D. Ubiquitin

24. Barr body is found in the following phase of the cell cycle:
A. Interphase
B. Metaphase
C. GI phase
D. Telophase

25. Nitric oxide is produced in:
A. Endothelium
B. Plasma
C. Platelets
D. Serum

26. Nightmares are seen in:
A. REM sleep
B. NREM stage II
C. NREM stage IB
D. NREM stage IV

27. Hypoxia causes vasoconstriction in:
A. Muscle
B. Lungs
C. Liver
D. Spleen

28. Which one of the following is the correct sequence in increasing order of their basal blood supply (ml/min/l00g of tissue)?
A. Heart, brain, kidney
B. Brain, kidney, heart
C. Kidney, heart, brain
D. Brain, heart, kidney

29. In the adrenal gland, androgens are produced by the cells in the:
A. Zona glomerulosa
B. Zona reticularis
C. Zona fasciculatea
D. Medulla

30. Resting membrane potential on nerve is determined by concentration of:
A. Calcium
B. Potassium

C. Chloride
D. Magnesium

31. **Blood brain barrier is deficient at:**
A. Area postrema
B. Thalamus
C. Meta thalamus
D. Cerebellum

32. **Phagocytosis in the CNS is done by:**
A. Astrocytes
B. Schwann cells
C. Microglia
D. Oligocytes

33. **Ventilation perfusion ratio is maximum in:**
A. Base of lung
B. Apex of lung
C. Post lobe of lung
D. Middle lobe of lung

34. **The state of iron responsible for O_2 transport:**
A. Fe^{++}
B. Fe^{+++}
C. Both
D. None

35. **Lung diffusion capacity is measured with:**
A. CO_2
B. CO
C. O_2
D. H_2

36. **Destruction of lateral nucleus of hypothalamus lead to:**
A. Aphagia
B. Hyperphagia
C. Satiety
D. Somnolence

37. **Milk ejection reflex is mediated by the hormone:**
A. Oxytocin
B. Vasopressin
C. Growth hormone
D. Thyroxin

38. The anterior lobe of hypophysis secretes the following *except:*

A. Somatotrophic hormone
B. Prolactin
C. Thyrotrophic hormone
D. Antidiuretic hormone

39. The affinity of oxygen for Hb decreases with fall in pH. This is called:

A. Brain bridge effect
B. Bhor effect
C. Haldane effect
D. Herring effect

40. Right shift of oxygen dissociation curve occurs in all *except*:

A. Transfusion
B. Shock
C. RDS
D. CHF

41. Injection of hypertonic saline into which area causes diuresis:

A. Supraoptic nucleus
B. Paraventricular nucleus
C. Preoptic nucleus
D. Posterior pituitary

42. Capillaries with tight junctions allowing the passage of only small molecules are found in:

A. Brain
B. Skin
C. Kidney
D. Muscle

43. The frequency of α wave an EEG is:

A. 18-30/s
B. 4-6/s
C. 8-12/s
D. 12-14/s

44. Chemical gradient across cell membrane is maintained chiefly by:

A. Na+
B. Ca + +
C. K +
D. Cl-

45. Action potentials are produced by:
A. Na^+ Influx
B. Na^+ -K^+ Influx
C. K^+ Influx
D. K^+ Efflux

46. Pain producing substance is:
A. Serotonin
B. Substance P
C. Histamine
D. Acetyl choline

47. The band which disappears on muscle contraction is:
A. I
B. H
C. A
D. Z

48. Blood flow in ml/100g/min is maximum in:
A. Kidneys
B. Liver
C. Heart
D. Skin

49. The organ with maximum O_2 consumption ml per minute:
A. Liver
B. Brain
C. Skeletal muscle
D. Heart

50. Calcium binding protein is:
A. Troponin C
B. Calsecritin
C. Calsequestrin
D. All

51. Red colour blindness is called:
A. Duteranopia
B. Protanopia
C. Protanomaly
D. Duteranomaly

52. Most common colour blindness is:
A. Duteranopia
B. Protanopia
C. Protanomaly
D. Duteranomaly

53. Delta waves in EEG are seen in:

A. Deep sleep
B. Rem sleep
C. Awake with eyes open
D. Awake with eyes closed

54. The freezing point of normal human plasma is:

A. 4°C
B. 0°C
C. -0.54°C
D. -4°C

ANSWERS

1. **C.** Polyspike and wave
2. **D.** Renal
3. **D.** Calcium binds to tropomyosin to initiate muscle contraction
4. **C.** Gate controlled theory of pain
5. **B.** Hyperactivity
6. **A.** Diastolic blood pressure
7. **A.** Sertoli and sertoli cells
8. **C.** Prevention of Ca2+ influx
9. **B.** Immediately increase in venous return to heart):
10. **C.** Occurs after follicular ripening by FSH
11. **A.** Contain serotonin
12. **A.** For passive diffusion down the concentration gradient
13. **A.** Epsilon and zeta
14. **D.** Intractable seizures
15. **C.** Damage to both respiratory apparatus and respiratory centre):
16. **D.** Mollusc shell
17. **A.** Lateral movement of proteins
18. **A.** Protanomaly
19. **B.** Decrease in K+ permeability
20. **C.** 7 cal
21. **D.** Shift in the oxygen dissociation curve to the left
22. **D.** Glutamate
23. **D.** Ubiquitin
24. **A.** Interphase
25. **A.** Endothelium
26. **A.** REM sleep
27. **B.** Lungs
28. **D.** Brain, heart, kidney
29. **B.** Zona reticularis
30. **B.** Potassium
31. **A.** Area postrema
32. **C.** Microglia
33. **B.** Apex of lung
34. **A.** Fe^{++}
35. **B.** CO

36. **A.** Aphagia
37. **A.** Oxytocin
38. **D.** Antidiuretic hormone
39. **B.** Bhor effect
40. **A.** Transfusion: Because the amount of 2,3 DPG in stored blood is reduced. In all other conditions there is acidosis.
41. **A.** Supraoptic nucleus
42. **A.** Brain
43. **C.** 8-12/s
44. **C.** K +
45. **A.** Na+ Influx
46. **B.** Substance P
47. **B.** H
48. **A.** Kidneys
49. **A.** Liver
50. **A.** Troponin C
51. **B.** Protanopia
52. **D.** Duteranomaly
53. **A.** Deep sleep
54. **C.** -0.54°C